the PERVERSION
of AUTONOMY

coercion and constraints in a liberal society

Willard Gaylin & Bruce Jennings

Georgetown University Press
Washington, D.C.

Georgetown University Press, Washington, D.C.
© 2003 by Georgetown University Press. All rights reserved.
Printed in the United States of America

10   9   8   7   6   5   4   3   2   1   2003

This volume is printed on acid-free offset book paper.

Library of Congress Cataloging-in-Publication Data

Gaylin, Willard.
    The perversion of autonomy : coercion and constraints in a liberal
society / Willard Gaylin, Bruce Jennings.—Revised and expanded.
        p. cm.
Includes bibliographical references and index.
    ISBN 0-87840-906-8 (pbk : alk. paper)
    1. Individualism—United States. 2. Libertarianism—United States.
3. Civil society—United States. 4. Social ethics—United States.
5. Involuntary treatment—United States. I. Jennings, Bruce, 1949–
II. Title.
JC599.US   G36   2003
320.51'2—dc21

                                                    2002013910

To Dr. Irene Crowe
with affection and gratitude for your longstanding
encouragement and support

To the memory of
Hugh J. Jennings and Margaret E. Jennings
for the past

And to Andrew M. Jennings
for the future

Contents

Preface

WHAT DOES IT mean to be free? What constraints on freedom are legitimate in the service of social living? These are the questions we addressed in 1996 in the first edition. These questions have an added sense of urgency since September 11, 2001.

There is no escaping the fact that the America we wrote about several years ago is not the same America we seek to fathom today. Almost overnight, people came to look upon government with a newfound admiration and sense of resolve. The 1990s had been a time of remarkable prosperity and had seemed to many a time of endless, petty political bickering and backbiting. The presidential election of 2000 was one of the most divisive and bitter in American history. With the assault on our homeland, the alienation and disgust seemed to disappear. People once divided came together in a sense of common purpose. The same people who had burned flags during the Vietnam era were now displaying them in the windows of their SUVs, BMWs, or Ford Escorts.

Within a few days after the attack, Attorney General John Ashcroft went before Congress to argue for a sweeping new law, the Anti-Terrorism Act of 2001, that would, in effect, defend life and liberty by considerably increasing the power of the federal government to investigate and to intrude in the telecommunications and financial transactions of private citizens. The attorney general spoke of a balance between the capabilities of law enforcement in an era when terrorists command sophisticated global telecommunications capabilities and traditional constitutional and civil liberties.

Noted civil libertarian and constitutional scholar Laurence Tribe of Harvard University soon added his voice to the discussion of balancing by pointing out that individual rights could not trump everything; the Constitution was never meant to be a suicide pact for the society. Nonetheless, he was also somewhat reserved and leery about the willingness of Congress and the Supreme Court to achieve the correct balance. What most concerned him was the temptation of the American people, in this time of danger, fear, and anger, to accept too many restrictions and to accept a kind of government power that the Constitution ought to prohibit.

As we gained more distance from the shock of September 11, it became clear that although some attitudes and assumptions had changed, more fundamental values and expectations had not. It turns out that we were not susceptible to the siren's song of authority, order, and coercion after all. The Constitution seems secure even with a conservative Supreme Court, and will not be easily or quickly shredded, as many libertarian activists feared. The painstaking work of balancing rights and responsibilities in our public life will go on, like the slow drilling of hard wood.

In fashioning the second edition of *The Perversion of Autonomy* we have retained the main body of the original, although thoroughly revising and updating it. We recognize now—even more than originally—how crucial developments in health, medicine, and the biomedical sciences have been in fostering and shaping the culture of autonomy during the last half of the last century. We have added, therefore, two chapters on medical care at the end of life that further amplify our sense of human interdependency through the cycle of life. At first blush, it would seem that if maximal respect for autonomy is going to be morally compelling and socially workable anywhere, it will be in the final weeks and months of a dying person's life. One of the culture of autonomy's strongest manifestations since the first edition of this book has been the movement to legalize physician-assisted suicide, and the attempt to make euthanasia morally acceptable. It turns out that even at the end of life autonomy does not function well as the overriding value, and does not provide an adequate moral vision to guide our public policies or our personal responsibilities.

In 1996, some of our conservative friends were disappointed by the fact that we did not use our energies to bash liberalism, but instead tried to revivify it with a more communal and civic sensibility; and some of our liberal friends felt that we had given too much of the "self" away in defense of community. We hope that our efforts may strike a more responsive chord in the climate of this current decade.

Acknowledgments

ALTHOUGH ONLY ABOUT fifteen months in the writing, this book has been closer to fifteen years in the making. Those were years of collaboration between the authors and their many colleagues at The Hastings Center, where careful and passionate argument about autonomy, coercion, community, and goodness is literally a daily occurrence.

In a more immediate sense this work grew out of a project at The Hastings Center on the ethics of coercion and social control, supported by the Pettus-Crowe Foundation in 1993–94. The participants in that project gave us much that we have drawn upon, and we would like to acknowledge Irene Crowe, Strachan Donnelley, James Nelson, Hilde Nelson, Philip Boyle, Mark Hanson, Bette Crigger, Erik Parens, Richard Hull, Michael Rhodes, Claudia Mills, John Arras, and Bonnie Steinbock. Early drafts of portions of the book were read by Aryeh Botwinick, Irene Crowe, Betty Gaylin, Maggie Jennings, Mildred Solomon, and Ronald Bayer, and we thank them for their help.

Charles Taylor gave us some useful guidance while he was Hans Jonas Visiting Scholar at The Hastings Center. Judith Audre, E. Fuller Torrey, Thomas Szasz, and others have spoken or written publicly on the first edition of the book, and we have tried to benefit from their criticisms.

The late Erwin A. Glikes, master editor and friend, gave us the early resolve to see this project through by his enthusiastic sense that our topic was a vital and timely one. Shortly before his death in 1994, Erwin brought us to The Free Press, where we have had the good fortune to work with Susan Arellano. Her careful reading and thoughtful suggestions have improved the book from start to finish, and we are most grateful to her. Our literary agent, Owen Laster, also provided support and encouragement that were extremely helpful and greatly appreciated. Richard Brown of Georgetown University Press breathed new life into the book by encouraging us to revise, update, and expand it for a second edition. Buoyed by his enthusiasm and guided by his suggestions, we have produced a work intended as a look forward toward a new moral sensibility in our culture, no less than as a critical reading of fin-de-siècle America.

We would like to acknowledge a special debt of gratitude to Daniel Callahan, president and cofounder of The Hastings Center, who has been a constant source of stimulating ideas and rigorous thinking about fundamental ethical issues for both of us for many years. His has been a pioneering voice in social ethics questioning the primacy of autonomy.

Research and administrative support were provided by Jennifer Stuber, Mary Ann Hasbrouck, Janet Bower, and Marna Howarth. We are most grateful to them.

In writing this book the importance of families has never been far from our minds, and our own families have provided patience, criticism, and support. Our wives, Betty Gaylin and Maggie Jennings, have served us with love and support in this project as in all other aspects of our lives. We are grateful to them and for them.

This book is dedicated to Irene Crowe. Sponsor, critic, colleague, and all-around good friend, she has at various times encouraged, prodded, induced, seduced, and cajoled us to the completion of this project. She is truly coauthor of this effort.

I

Freedom, Coercion, and Commonsense Morality

> Some philosophers ... seem to think that the question "Do you believe that the earth has existed for many years past?" is not a plain question, such as should be met either by a plain "Yes" or "No," ... but is the sort of question which can be properly met by: "It all depends on what you mean by 'the earth' and 'exists' and 'years': if you mean so and so, and so and so, and so and so, then I do; but if you mean so and so, and so and so, and so and so, ... I think it is extremely doubtful." It seems to me that such a view is as profoundly mistaken as any view can be.
>
> —G. E. Moore, "A Defense of Common Sense"

AN AMERICAN TRAGEDY

William Black, a fifty-five-year-old homeless man, lived with his friends Bobby Tunkins and Lala Wigfall under the scaffolding at 113th Street and Amsterdam Avenue in Manhattan, just across the street from St. Luke's Hospital. They made their living scavenging cans and bottles and collecting the deposit money. A good day would bring in ten dollars and keep them stocked with beer and wine.

Pop, as his friends called him, was born in Baltimore, the son of a steelworker. As an adult he held various jobs, and he was married, with two children. In the mid-1970s he became unemployed, started drinking, and had some trouble with the law. His marriage broke up. In 1977 he moved to New York to work in a factory with his younger brother. In 1980 the factory closed. Life went downhill for Pop Black after that, and by the late eighties he was living on the streets.

1

On the morning of October 17, 1994, Mr. Black was making his rounds collecting cans when he complained of feeling achy and began to cough up blood. By late that afternoon he was too sick to move, so Mr. Tunkins left him sitting on a sidewalk grate and went across the street to the hospital to get help. There he was informed that hospital policy prevented any doctors or nurses from leaving the emergency room. "That would be counterproductive to the mission of the ER, confusing and a waste of time," a hospital spokesperson later said. Tunkins was told to call 911. An ambulance responded about seven minutes later.

At this point stories conflict. Tunkins believes that Black was delirious and did not know where he was or what he was saying. The EMS technicians believed that Black was lucid and reported that he refused medical assistance. They left him where he was. "We don't have a mechanism in place to force someone to go to the hospital," an EMS official said later. "He was an RMA—refused medical attention."

Shortly after seven o'clock the next morning Mr. Tunkins and Ms. Wigfall found Pop Black unconscious and called EMS again. After some delay the ambulance crew arrived and pronounced him dead at 7:37 A.M. But they still did not pick him up; other arms of the city bureaucracy are in charge of that. Normally a dead body on the street is removed as quickly as possible in New York City. However, that morning was a busy one and Pop Black lay on the sidewalk in death for four hours, as he had done for the final fifteen hours of his life. "The thing about William," his brother told a reporter from the *New York Times*, "was that he fell from grace." Just so. However, his autonomy, his right to RMA, was respected to the end.[1]

William Black stands for many things. He was a casualty of what is so innocently called the "restructuring of the job market" that wreaks havoc in many communities and many lives in the United States today. He was also a casualty of the alcohol and drug abuse that is sapping the vitality of our society like a spreading cancer. Whether due to a mental illness or simply to a personal inability to cope with hard times, he became a statistic not only of unemployment but also of homelessness. Yet he also showed, from what little we can tell, that life on the street has its friendships, its loyalties, and its pleasures. The Nazis would have called him "life unworthy of life," but that is a monstrous, evil notion. Our own morality is put to the test precisely by unfortunates like William Black—by those who reach out in need of help, in need of rescue (perhaps even from themselves), and who morally demand a response.

Did we fail this test? William Black's story is particularly significant because it symbolizes one of the deepest moral and emotional divisions of our time. Virtually everyone to whom we have told this story responds with shock and sadness. A moral common sense, we believe, is still widespread in America, and it reacts almost viscerally to situations like this. Common sense tells us to reach out to those in need, to step up and take charge of a situation when we can clearly see disaster impending or needless hurt coming. Of course William Black should have been given medical attention. Of course the hospital across the street should have been open to him, and someone, somehow should have gotten him there. Of course.

On the other hand, many people we have talked to about this incident shake their heads ruefully and say that they can understand exactly how this kind of thing happens. They appreciate the pathos of Pop Black, but they think the EMS policy of letting individuals who refuse medical assistance alone is the best the city can do. They recognize that paternalism is a dangerous thing, especially when officials of the state, like EMS workers, exercise power over adults, supposedly for their own good.

What are EMS officials to do? They encounter strange, irrational, self-destructive behavior every day. Common sense can be overwhelmed by circumstances. In this case, the public policy response is to err on the side of a person's autonomy, even if the foreseeable result is that a person who could have been saved will die. Moral common sense is exasperated by that response—considers it a scandal, an outrage.

Moral common sense would have us reach out to help, to do what it *knows* is right, without the nitpicking and quibbles that so exasperated G. E. Moore. It respects the humanity of others by sensing connectedness with them and with their vulnerability.

In our society the counterbalancing current to this moral common sense is respect for the personal liberty of the individual. This liberty consists in the right to live your own life in your own way; in the words of Justice Louis Brandeis, it is the right to be let alone. William Black's life was not unworthy of life; his humanity was not unworthy of respect, concern, and care from others. But then, neither was his life unworthy of freedom.

THE CULTURE OF AUTONOMY

The moral crosscurrents in America today are complex. This book is about the intersection of interdependence and autonomy, of individual rights and mutual responsibility. A natural sensibility impels us to see ourselves in relationships of interdependence with other people and to take responsibility both for our own lives and for what happens to others as well. We are our brothers' keepers. Cain lacked this sensibility; most Americans possess it, so far. At the same time, we have a powerful and valuable tradition of personal liberty and respect for rights, privacy, and independence. Individuals need the elbow room that respect for autonomy provides in order to grow, express themselves, pursue their own goals, and yes, even make their own mistakes.

Common sense often tells us to intervene, get involved, use persuasion, inducements, pressure, or coercion, if necessary, to turn a bad situation around, to stave off foreseeable evil. However, respect for autonomy often tells us not to interfere and not to use the multiple resources of influence and coercion that culture and psychology put at our disposal.

There is wisdom in both responses. Often we have to make a hard choice between them. Two extremes we must avoid: We must avoid paralysis, indecision, and moral drift, and we must avoid systematically opting for one of these values to the virtual exclusion of the other. Our thesis in this book is that the morality of interdependence and mutual responsibility has been clashing with respect for autonomy with increasing frequency and harshness for the past thirty years, and that autonomy has won in these clashes too often. Reason does not require that autonomy be abandoned, only that its balance with other individual and communal values be restored.

Autonomy's success in the struggle for the American moral imagination has made it overbearing and overweening. When obeisance to personal liberty and independence triumphs systematically over a relational, communitarian commonsense morality, then a set of attitudes, unexamined assumptions, and a political and ethical style and rhetoric develop that we shall refer to as the "culture of autonomy."

This book is about that culture of autonomy, its appeal, its excesses, and its limits. Drawing on many examples of domestic life and social policy, we aim to put the culture of autonomy in a more balanced and critical perspective. We shall explore where it came from, its philosophical underpinnings (part I); its biological and psychological limits (part II); and the moral, social, and political dangers it poses (part III). In these days when respect for the communist state has long since disappeared from even the most deluded fellow traveler, it may seem perverse to criticize the individualism that has served liberal democracy so well. But freed of the political dialectic of the cold war, it may be easier for us now to perceive the danger inherent in the distortion and exaggeration of our society's core values, especially one as crucial as personal liberty or autonomy.

The reader might well wonder why we single out the concept of "autonomy" for special emphasis and attention. To some extent the choice is arbitrary for it does not mean only one thing but connotes a rich cluster of related but subtly distinct ideas. We will try to sort out and explain that cluster of ideas in chapter 2, although even that discussion is too brief to do full justice to the concept and is no substitute for the kind of careful scholarship exemplified by Jerome Schneewind's definitive work.[2] Moreover, there are several very similar or virtually equivalent notions that have been the focus of important studies by leading social theorists and social scientists. For example, our analysis of the culture of autonomy overlaps in many ways with what historian Christopher Lasch called the "culture of narcissism." It has affinities as well with what philosopher Charles Taylor has referred to as the "ethics of authenticity." Robert Bellah and his colleagues called it "expressive individualism." Finally, at the heart of what we are concerned with under the heading of autonomy is a notion that sociologist Alan Wolfe has called "moral freedom."[3] He defines his subject in the following way:

> The old adage that America is a free country has, at last, come true, for Americans have come to accept the relevance of individual freedom, not only in their economic and political life, but in their moral life as well. The defining characteristic of the moral philosophy of the Americans can therefore be described as the principle of moral freedom. Moral freedom means that individuals should determine for themselves what it means to lead a good and virtuous life. Contemporary Americans find answers to the perennial questions asked by theologians and moral philosophers, not by conforming to strictures handed down by God or nature, but by considering who they are, what others require, and what consequences follow from acting

one way rather than another. Some of our respondents adopt moral freedom as a creative challenge. . . . [T]hey find themselves quite comfortable with the idea that a good society is one that allows each individual maximum scope for making his or her own moral choices.[4]

Wolfe goes on to argue that the widespread (but by no means universal) embrace of moral freedom amounts to a cultural revolution in America: "never have so many people been so free of moral constraint as contemporary Americans. Most people, throughout most of the world, have lived under conditions in which their morality was defined for them. Now, for the first time in human history, significant numbers of individuals believe that people should play a role in defining their own morality as they contemplate their proper relationship to God, to one another, and to themselves."[5]

Self-sovereignty in the moral realm; the right to live your own life in your own way so long as you do others no harm; being true to yourself above all—these notions are at the core of individualism, authenticity, moral freedom, and autonomy, if not as all professional philosophers would define them, then at least as many ordinary Americans define them in their own social and self-consciousness. Wolfe is relatively sanguine about the effects of the cultural influence of moral freedom; we are less so about the culture of autonomy. The dark side of the culture of autonomy is becoming increasingly apparent: something akin to decadence is setting in. Individualism, privacy, and rights claims are sometimes so overblown that they become caricatures of themselves. The individualistic philosophy that has been the backbone of political liberalism and that protects the person from the power of the state has become hyperextended into a kind of libertarian liberalism that sees power, and nothing but power, everywhere, and that casts the same acids of suspicion and mistrust on the family and civil associations that political liberals have traditionally reserved for the government.

Extending the claims of autonomy as America has been doing recently is dangerous for two reasons. First, it invites a politically and socially reactionary backlash that could threaten civil liberties across the board, and not just the exaggerated ones. Equally dangerous, but more subtle and insidious, is the possibility that it will come to undermine the very social and psychic infrastructure upon which social order, and hence the conditions for autonomy itself, rests. The social infrastructure to which we refer consists primarily of the family and the various civic institutions through which individuals live as parents, friends, and neighbors; as church, synagogue, or mosque members; as volunteers, professionals, and citizens. The psychic infrastructure endangered by the culture of autonomy is those processes of childrearing, socialization, and moral development that create the motivational basis for responsible conduct in the social emotions of shame, guilt, pride, and conscience. Maintaining these foundations of social order requires respect for authority as well as respect for freedom; it requires institutional power and restraint as well as self-expression and independence.

The phase of decadent individualism that America seems to be entering is eroding the very humanity of the individuals whose freedom we are presuming to respect and to protect. Freedom, liberty, autonomy, choice, personal rights, voluntarism, and finally empowerment are now the most often used and revered words in our moral and civic discourse. They constitute the vocabulary, and support the syntax, of a specific political and moral discourse. Behind them stands a particular vision of what it means to be a human individual, a self, and a vision of what social relationships and arrangements ought to be to nurture that self. Together they support a theory that one "chooses" one's behavior voluntarily and that the conduct of others can generally be modified through rational argument—"Just say no."

This is simplistic, reflects an inadequate understanding of human motivation, and ultimately is philosophically and morally untenable. The perspective and position we develop in the following chapters is built around four central premises:

Human beings are products of their environment as well as their creators; therefore the sacrifice of the community for the sake of the individual is a no-win game. Protection of individual rights at the expense of a safe environment provides neither. The ghetto woman who is not free to leave her home unattended to do her nightly shopping in safety is not free.

Social controls are an essential aspect of any sustainable, viable society, including liberal and democratic ones. Yet just as the culture of autonomy has cast nearly all aspects of freedom in terms of personal liberty, rights, and independence, so too a pervasive libertarian rhetoric tars all aspects of social control with the brush of physical force, bodily invasion, and coercion. At more heated moments, there is a disturbing tendency to talk as though nothing exists between full autonomy and slavery, between complete independence and threats of violence, between total control of a situation and rape. Even in more restrained and thoughtful debates, autonomy is set up as the antithesis of coercion, and coercion the antithesis of autonomy, so that to the extent one is present, the other is absent. This autonomy/coercion polarity influences the debates on a vast host of social problems, from teenage pregnancy to foreign affairs, from genetic experimentation to drug abuse policy. Except in the minds of a few purists, the polarity was never originally intended to suggest a moral bias in favor of freedom and against coercion. Nonetheless, it has generally been viewed that way. The autonomy/coercion polarity is almost inevitably perceived as a "good guy/bad guy" polarity.

Coercion is not always bad, and it is not even always the enemy of autonomy, or at least of freedom in a somewhat broader sense. Civilization depends in great part on the right of the community to insist on certain conduct from its citizens. Given the social nature of human beings, our sheer individual survival depends on some limited social order. Human flourishing, the realization of our full moral and creative potential, requires a social order correspondingly complex.

The structure of organized society rests on defined limits of freedom. The law not only defines unacceptable behavior but also establishes punishments—coercive forces—that may be used to ensure compliance. Without those punishments, the law is as helpless as an unarmed prophet. Income tax and traffic laws are more likely to be obeyed in societies that punish offenders than in those that do not. Social order rests, in a liberal society no less than in a totalitarian one, on the use of coercion.

Human behavior is less "voluntary" than libertarians and theorists of autonomy would have it. Present behavior is significantly determined by past treatment. Modern psychology has only too clearly shown that the child we neglect, to whom we deny care, guidance, and comfort, will repay us by becoming an adult who is incapable of choosing to care and protect—or even respect—others.

Human behavior is less rational than most of us would like to believe it is. When it comes to changing conduct, appeals to the emotions are usually more effective than logical argument. Fear, greed, shame, guilt, and pride fuel the machinery of behavior. To motivate morally appropriate behavior, society is entitled to—indeed occasionally must—appeal to any or all of these emotions through its institutions, laws, and norms. Individuals often must do the same in their interactions with others. It is not immoral to utilize these effective methods for changing behavior for the good of society and the good of the individual. Persuasion, influence, inducement, seduction, rewards, threats, and even physical constraint—the entire spectrum of "social control"—comes into clearer moral focus when one understands the nature of the human being, the principles that influence conduct, and the interdependence of personhood and culture.

THE TRANSFORMATION OF FREEDOM INTO AUTONOMY

Despite an enormous body of psychological knowledge of motivation, our leaders and our public policies continue to aspire to a radically voluntary society, a social order based virtually on rational will and voluntary consent alone. This voluntary society would impose no legal or moral requirements that are not ultimately rooted in the concepts of autonomy and consent.

Yet the products of this world of "freedom" are disturbing:

- The mentally ill and the addicted are left like so much refuse on the desolate and dangerous streets of our urban centers. Homeless men and women cannot be taken to shelters (or even to hospitals) by city officials "against their will." The arrogance of autonomy allows them the freedom to freeze to death on city streets.

- After hitting record highs in the late 1980s and early 1990s, the number of teenage pregnancies has declined but unwanted pregnancy and single-parent families remain problems. In the national debate the notion of "reproductive rights" is often appealed to, but "reproductive responsibility" is ridiculed as a code word for the coercion of women and minorities. Thus, a young woman, without reproductive counseling or contraceptive services, is "free" to get pregnant; "free" to rear her children in poverty; and "free" to remain uneducated, thus dooming herself and her child to membership in what is becoming a permanent underclass.

- Newborn babies born with AIDS could be helped by early treatment, but identifying and treating them is hindered by our obsession with rights of privacy. Such treatment would require, in effect, testing and notifying the mother (because no newborn is HIV-positive without the mother being so too), thus violating the mother's right to keep her own condition secret. If she remains ignorant of her own condition, she may infect other partners and deprive herself of beneficial treatments. So be it if privacy is the transcendent principle of our society. But what kind of society is it that allows babies to be born doomed to disease and death when we have an effective treatment at hand?

Such are the fruits of the culture of autonomy. But in protecting such autonomy are we really enhancing freedom? We intuitively know that the teenage crack addict is not a "free" human being, even if we assume—naïvely—that because she took the crack without any coercion, she voluntarily chose to become a user. Moreover, we must ask if teenage pregnancy, defended as a right to be protected from the slightest suggestion of coercion, actually serves freedom. It certainly can hobble reasonable efforts to protect and promote senses of freedom that autonomy has forgotten. When a Planned Parenthood group effectively offered a dollar-a-day to teenage girls who protected themselves from pregnancy, the program—which was surprisingly effective—was nonetheless attacked as coercive.

A too-rigid defense of autonomy interferes with more sophisticated concepts of freedom. It is hard to imagine a paranoid schizophrenic living in the streets of New York, or a drug addict, as being a "free agent." When logical analysis leads to conclusions that affront the common sense of a vast majority of knowledgeable people, their common sense must be respected. What must be examined is the "logic" underlying the contradicting analysis.

Examples such as these are not quirks or marginal instances of extreme views. They generally represent what is becoming *the* vision of America: a vision of the autonomous self in a voluntary society. How has autonomy come to triumph in this way? A definitive and thorough historical explanation of this development has not yet emerged, although aspects of the problem that we have found helpful and suggestive can be found in works by David Riesman, Robert Bellah and colleagues, and E. J. Dionne.[6] In any case, the task we have set ourselves in this book is less to explain the culture of autonomy than to take its moral pulse and to diagnose its underlying blind spots and misconceptions. Nor will we attempt to document or demonstrate the pervasiveness of autonomy in some empirical or social scientific way. We offer instead an interpretation based on observation and examples drawn from the world of everyday life that will be, we hope, familiar to most readers.

The problem with the culture of autonomy is that its vision is not working and can never work. As a vision of America, it is profoundly mistaken, tragically flawed. It is increasingly untenable and damaging as a guiding principle. It cannot define what is most valuable in our lives, how we come to be who we are, or how society must be arranged to promote both the individual and the common good.

Americans have embraced freedom so tightly, they can now see only one aspect of it, the side of autonomy. However, freedom has many faces and has carried many meanings in the Western cultural tradition. For Pericles in ancient Athens, it meant self-confidence, vitality, and being in charge of one's own affairs. This is a spirit that lets a person—or a whole society—be open to the world, and to absorb it, without getting lost in it. For Saint Paul, perfect freedom was perfect servitude, albeit in the service of Christ.

Aristotle thought that political freedom consisted in ruling and being ruled in turn. Otantes, another ancient Greek, found freedom in neither ruling nor being ruled. Abraham Lincoln shared this latter sentiment: as he would not be another man's slave, neither would he enslave another man.

For the English political philosopher Thomas Hobbes, freedom meant the absence of external restraint necessary to impede even destructive passions of individual will, whereas for his successor in the development of liberal thought, John Locke, it meant security of person and possessions in a society of shared laws and reasonable expectations. Jean-Jacques Rousseau, by contrast, thought that selfishness actually enslaves us and that there is no contradiction in saying that sometimes people must be "forced to be free." Mandatory education for all children is a corollary of this thesis.

Heirs to all these visions of freedom and more, we modern men and women in the Western world stake much of our self-identity and civic pride on them. When we talk of freedom in our public discourse, it is with worshipful and unexamined awe. It is therefore particularly disturbing to recognize that in trying to pay homage to freedom, we are in fact disfiguring it.

The ideals of self and society and the experiences captured by the term *autonomy* are one, but only one, set of the ideals and experiences that historically and psychologically can be captured under the idea of freedom. Autonomy, understood as independence, freedom of choice, and the right to be left alone, is an important facet of freedom, but it is not the only important one. When autonomy walks alone and tries to do all the moral work that a more complex understanding of freedom should do, it stumbles. A single-minded preoccupation with autonomy has already blinded us to some states of affairs that truly threaten freedom, in the broader, more communal sense of the term. Poverty and ignorance can restrict freedom of action as effectively as restrictive legislation, and perhaps more.

This returns us to the simplistic polarity between autonomy and coercion, where autonomy is always the "good guy" and coercion is always bad, forgetting in the process that coercion is an essential component of social control and a necessary means of maintaining social order, upon which freedom itself depends. When voluntary persuasion fails and only coercion works, and when it serves both the public and the individual good, coercion can be morally justified. Public health measures such as infectious-disease control and mandatory vaccination programs for children are paradigmatic examples of justified coercion.

COMMONSENSE MORALITY AND THE LIMITS OF AUTONOMY

Freedom and coercion have been central concerns of both authors through their involvement with the work of The Hastings Center, a private research institute studying ethical and social issues in medicine and the life sciences founded in 1969. A meeting ground for philosophers, sociologists, constitutional and criminal lawyers, physicians, biologists, theologians, and others, its concern was (and still is) the ethical dilemmas emerging from the rapidly evolving technologies of biology and medicine. These advances suggested that an agenda of unprecedented issues would soon emerge, including the definition of death, test-tube babies, genetic engineering, organ transplants, human behavior control and modification, population control, suicide, and the right to die. This agenda would demand a new consideration of old and neglected moral principles.

To launch our interdisciplinary effort into what has since become known as "bioethics," one of the first research groups organized at the Center was a task force on freedom and coercion. We correctly anticipated that this would be a pivotal issue underlying future debates in medical ethics.

But surely the context and time of our beginnings were important. In the late 1960s the concept of freedom was on everyone's mind. The United States was fighting a miserable war that was increasingly tearing American society asunder, raising critical questions about national purpose. Young were pitted against old, affluent against poor, all in the name of "freedom" and democracy—a familiar stance for Americans.

We were battling against the totalitarian evil of a repressive and coercive communist world. Most of us then perceived freedom in terms of the splendid and isolated individual protecting his or her sacred autonomy against the tyranny of an oppressive state, later captured in the emblematic image of the lonely hero in Tiananmen Square placing his body and his life in the path of a column of tanks.

Of course, coercion was also woven into the fabric of our society. Under penalty of law, society still forces infants to be inoculated against childhood infectious diseases. It forces children to attend school. It forces workers to save a part of their earnings through the conditions of the Social Security Act. The law forces people to attain licensure in order to drive, and later to use seat belts or helmets. And society forced people, via the draft, to risk their lives in the service of their country.

Perhaps it was partly the reaction against military conscription during an unpopular war that made Americans lose sight of those justified mandatory requirements, including civic service and limitations on the pursuit of self-interest, that are essential in a free and liberal society. At any rate, so lost were these threads of humane coercion in the overall libertarian pattern of the 1960s and later that they ceased to be identified for what they were. If it was "freedom" we were fighting for in the jungles of Southeast Asia, then it was "freedom" that we would fight for—with a vengeance—in the United States in the late 1960s and early 1970s.

The Hastings Center was formed not to fight that battle but to examine the sociology, psychology, and morality of health and illness. The venue for these battles is not the street or the jailhouse but homes and hospitals. The adversaries here are not the all-powerful state versus the beleaguered individual; the conflicts (if that is even the most appropriate word) are between mother and daughter, physician and patient, hospital and the physician, and (at its most political) the privileges of the affluent versus the needs of the indigent.

The concept of autonomy, the various definitions and meanings of which will be discussed more fully in chapters 2 and 3, means essentially that one makes one's own rules or choices. But does the senile, demented, or drugged person represent the true self, the real person? Although autonomy and freedom are related, they have different implications, and their ideas are contested in different arenas. The consequences of these distinctions are enormous.

Consider the following example. Several years ago we both attended a working conference on the ethical and political implications of the use of Norplant. Norplant is a system of long-term contraception that involves the surgical insertion of small rods containing a slow-release hormone under the skin of a woman's upper arm. This system allows for the slow release of small doses of a progestin (levonorgestral) into the woman's body and is capable of preventing pregnancy for up to five years. The rods may be removed at any time, but inserting and removing them involves a minor surgical procedure. Norplant was perceived by its developers as a safe and effective means to enable effective family planning and to promote reproductive freedom for women. Others did not see it that way.

The case under discussion at the conference was a Baltimore experiment in which Norplant was to be offered at a high school–based reproductive health clinic run by the city health department. The high school to pilot the program was largely made up of African-American students. A group of high school girls—with the approval of their families and with the cooperation of the school administrators—had indicated their desire to use the Norplant system. However, they were stymied by a political coalition of African American ministers and other community leaders who said that the girls were being "intimidated" or "coerced" into this action. These ministers felt that the "community" had not been adequately involved. They then launched an attack on the Norplant project, labeling it "racist," "genocidal," "human experimentation," and "coercive"; an infringement on the "freedom" and "autonomy" of the young women. This attack effectively sank the program.

The conversations around the table at the conference were heated, and they revealed something important about the shape and tenor of our current public discourse concerning autonomy. The discussants were largely women sophisticated in the language and science of women's reproduction, or veterans of the struggle for women's reproductive freedom. These same women had consistently argued, in the interminable public debates over abortion, that a pregnant woman's decision over her body was hers and hers alone. Not her husband's, not her boyfriend's, not her parents', not her minister's, and certainly not her community's. To our surprise, these same women, incredibly, took a different position in the case of Norplant. They opposed the Baltimore health department's program and sided with the community leaders.

Many of these women—in defense of pure autonomy—had actually worked actively *against* the Freedom of Choice Act (FOCA), which would have granted women the legislated right to abortion on demand—because the only act then passable was a compromise that would have included a twenty-four– to forty-eight–hour waiting period and/or some form of parental consent. They abandoned 99 percent of their program to defend the inviolability of their guiding principle of autonomy. This was a political decision to which they were entitled.

These same women who were totally committed to "unrestricted autonomy" where abortion is concerned—seemed to lose their fervor for autonomy in the Norplant debate and inconsistently began to speak the language of beneficence and paternalism.

They then proposed restrictions on services offering Norplant that *they themselves* would have rejected as outrageous and offensive if the word *abortion* had been substituted for *Norplant*. Reacting to these arguments, someone had the temerity to remind the participants that they might soon be confronted with state initiatives defining abortion rights, if the national protection of abortion rights were to be rescinded by Congress or the Supreme Court. "Are you proposing," they were asked, "that somehow or other abortion is a more trivial, less definitive or invasive procedure than the implantation of Norplant?" They were not. "Would you want these same guidelines adopted for abortion?" They certainly would not.

The participants were trapped in the contradictions of their own position. They viewed the Baltimore program as an intrusion on the "freedom" of these teenage girls, representing "coercive infringement of their autonomous rights." When it was pointed out that nothing had been mandated by the city government or by law, that Norplant would only be used "voluntarily," the participants expressed distrust for the "educative" methods that might be used. Even "persuasive" argument was defined as coercive rather than educative. The potential abuses of power and authority that are only too evident in the historic treatment of minority groups biased all debate.

The day after this meeting, a healthy infusion of commonsense morality was introduced into the debate by the then Surgeon General of the United States, Dr. Joycelyn Elders. Dr. Elders stated that young girls with unwanted pregnancies are in a condition of slavery: "If you're poor and ignorant, with a child, you're a slave. Meaning that you're never going to get out of it. These women are in bondage to a kind of slavery that the Thirteenth Amendment just didn't deal with."[7]

Dr. Elders—no philosopher, but an African American woman and a physician of wisdom and compassion—declared that teenage mothers are effectively deprived of their freedom as American citizens. Dr. Elders supports the use of Norplant as a *liberating* factor from the veritable "slavery" of teenage pregnancy.

To the uninitiated, Dr. Elders's common sense would seem to carry the day. How could having two, three, or four unwanted pregnancies during the time when one is supposed to be learning geography, history, and basic arithmetic enhance one's emergence into adulthood as an autonomous individual? For teenage girls, the "freedom" to become pregnant would seem inevitably to lead to a limitation of autonomy. We see the awful confusion that exists when autonomy is not clearly defined, when freedom is multiply defined, and when the two are not distinguished.

The assumption that "getting pregnant" is a free choice for a teenage girl is only one proposition against which we propose to test our definitions of freedom and coercion—a philosophical and psychological problem that has confounded the national debate in more areas than just pregnancy. The contradictions are worth examining.

Society's commitment to autonomy and freedom—even the definitions of rights, paternalism, coercion, choice—seems to fluctuate with changes in the political agenda. Although priorities may often change, definitions ought not to vary with political need. We must know, if not where we stand, at least what we are talking about.

HUMAN MOTIVATION AND THE LIMITS OF EDUCATION

One of the more astonishing features of current political debates on autonomy and coercion is the naïve underlying assumption about rationality and human motivation. Psychology—whether based on behaviorism or on its diametric opposite and antagonist, Freudianism (or on any of the splinters of these two dominant branches)—views few pieces of human conduct as rational choices selected at the moment. Rather, modern motivational psychology tends to see most human behavior as being "conditioned" or "unconsciously determined," a consequence or product of life experiences that tend to make given responses to certain stimuli automatic and unchosen.

This not-quite-reflexive behavior serves efficiency and is a substitute for the instinctual fixation of lower animals. Suppose, for example, three men are faced with the same mugger. They respond quite differently: one flees, one stands frozen in fear, and one attacks the mugger. These startlingly different responses cannot be explained on the basis of a rational analysis of the mugging situation. Rather, they express automatic yet different responses to the same stimulus when operating through a different perception, consciousness, and character—that is, a different *person* whose behavior and values have been shaped by past experiences of which he is often unaware.

Behavior that is set in the first few years of life is likely to be rigidly fixed and extraordinarily difficult to change later in life. In terms of moral conduct and social behavior, by the time we start the schooling of the average child, we have wasted our most precious opportunity to shape behavior, the first four years of life.

Some of the behavior conditioned in those first four years will take on the fixity and rigidity of instinct, forcing the emerging adult into certain predetermined patterns of behavior, for better or worse. This process limits the "freedom" or the autonomy of the individual in making many decisions that are normally seen as totally self-determined. There are times, indeed, when we are astounded at the irrationality of our own "decisions." The impulsive and emotional resistance of the intelligent and mature man or woman to the demands of the mugger who is about to take his or her money is usually recognized—even by the victim—as "stupid." However, certain lessons of childhood have set in motion impulses of behavior that compel even self-destructive action.

Not that psychologists have all the answers. Psychic determinism has in its own way gone too far, abandoning essential components of autonomy that *are* part of the human condition. The principle of a free (if only relatively free) individual underlies the notions of duty, obligation, and responsibility that are essential aspects of life in a free society.

To properly exercise our freedom, it may be that we must be "forced to be free" as Rousseau put it. We must guarantee the conditions of caring in childhood that alone can ensure the development of conscience, the capacity for guilt and shame, for empathy and generosity, for beneficence and identification—in other words, a moral sensibility.

SOURCES OF SELF-CONTROL

People tend to cling to their feelings of being totally autonomous. To do so, they often make some dangerous false assumptions about their own behavior. They deny the power of emotional influences on themselves, seeing themselves, if not others, as "rational" human beings. They prefer to see their failures and inadequacies as imposed from without or above— the fault lies in our stars, not within ourselves—whereas they will take full credit for their successes (that is, for having made the proper choices). Hence people are always more alert to dangers imposed on them by others— either by force or by manipulation—than to dangers emerging from self-determined behavior.

Take an example from the 1960s. Deep anxieties were emerging (later converted into a political crusade) concerning the effects of new technologies on the neurobiology of behavior. These technologies, with their presumed capacity to manipulate large populations of human beings, introduced a possibly new and frightening assault on human autonomy and political freedom. Subliminal advertising would reach deeply into our unconscious and manipulate us. Psychosurgery would create a class of human robots, an idea whose implementation was seriously considered by many of those who saw themselves as rational.

In the scientific community a serious debate in this area began with the flamboyant research of Dr. Jose Delgado.[8] By planting electrodes in the brains of animals, Dr. Delgado demonstrated his capacity to control the most violent and energetic behavior. With the flair of a natural-born media star, he showed how, by holding the proper instrument of control in his hand, he could stop a charging bull in midstride. Dr. Delgado and his charging bull were featured in all the newsmagazines of the day.

Subsequently, the possibility of electrode implantation as a means of controlling human behavior was introduced—not just by hysterics, the naïve, and political advocates looking for a cause, but by Dr. Delgado himself. He promised a golden future in which we could control such severe problems as "promiscuity in young girls" by electrical control of the human brain. Dr. Delgado himself might have passed unnoticed, but some eminently misguided neurologists, psychiatrists, and neurosurgeons at Harvard Medical School quickly jumped on the bandwagon he started. In order to attract interest in their own legitimate research on temporal lobe epilepsy (a decidedly unglamorous field), the Harvard researchers concluded that if they could generalize from *medical* control to social control, they might hit the funding jackpot.

Temporal lobe epilepsy has as one of its symptoms (as distinguished from the seizures associated with *grand mal* epilepsy) the capacity for irrational rages. The Harvard researchers decided that it might be propitious to link their research to the social discontent erupting during the Vietnam War. In the preface to a book directed to the general public, they linked the potential of their research on epilepsy to the control of riots in the inner cities, particularly Detroit, thereby discrediting themselves.[9]

In addition, at that time, psychiatry was considering what seemed to be the therapeutic potential of prefrontal lobotomy and psychosurgery. Prefrontal lobotomy was an overused and frighteningly oversold surgical procedure for controlling the behavior first of desperately ill psychotic patients and later of the not-so-desperately ill. With time we have come to realize that prefrontal lobotomy had very little potential for either good or bad. At the time, however, it was a natural focus for antiauthoritarian anxiety, and it became a dramatic subject for polemical theater. *Suddenly Last Summer* and *One Flew Over the Cuckoo's Nest* were only two of the very popular works that titillated and terrified the public.

The American public has a dangerous tendency to overvalue the threat of high-technology interventions (electrodes) and to undervalue the effects of low technology (television viewing). (This phenomenon has been labeled by Willard Gaylin as the "Frankenstein Factor."[10]) The major difference between implanting an electrode in the brain and implanting an idea is that it is generally easier to remove the electrode. The real danger for manipulating values and controlling behaviors, then as now, lies in the sixty-plus hours of television that the average four-year-old watches in any one week. It is easier to worry about electrodes, psychosurgery, and other externally imposed terrors than to worry about preschool education, family structure (or the lack thereof), and family responsibility in screening movie and television watching.

As individuals, our sense of worth and power is so tied to our need to see ourselves as free and autonomous agents that we will go to enormous extremes to protect that mythology. Unfortunately, we extend that narcissistic distortion beyond the individual and into the design of our institutions of education and policymaking. So frightened are we by communitarian beneficence, so staunchly protective of our individual rights, and so stubbornly libertarian, that we prefer to do that which is destined to fail—even when lives are at stake—rather than risk any assaults on our autonomy. We prefer to "educate" people, as though there were some mystery as to how AIDS is spread, how babies are born, how lung cancer is contracted, how bullets kill.

Consider the following extract, which appeared in summer 1994 in the *New York Times*:

> Federal auditors say a new Government program to distribute free vaccine to millions of children is plagued by serious problems, behind schedule, and will probably not increase immunization levels. Moreover, the auditors expressed doubt about a fundamental premise of the program: that the cost of vaccine is a major reason preschool children have not received the shots they need for protection against diseases like measles, mumps and polio. President Clinton persuaded Congress to establish the program in his first year in office by arguing that vaccine manufacturers were pursuing "profits at the expense of our children." But a report by the auditors of the General Accounting Office clearly indicated that "vaccine cost is not an important barrier" to the immunization of children. Indeed, the report stated, most children who are not vaccinated "are eligible for free vaccine under the present system."[11]

Public officials want to believe that parents are rational and logical. They like to think that if something essential to the safety and health of children is readily available and free, parents will avail themselves of it. So with the free vaccine, they assumed, all that was necessary would be to inform the population of its availability, and parents would take advantage of it.

There is something immoral about spending millions, even hundreds of millions, of dollars on programs to "educate" people to change their behavior, when we know that what is necessary is either intimidation or coercion.

Human behavior is never so simple or so rational as such policymakers hope. The same insight had to be discovered and rediscovered over a period of thirty years, in one political district after another. More than twenty years ago, New York City recognized that the majority of children in Harlem and other ghetto neighborhoods had not been vaccinated for polio. Free distribution was already in effect.

It was deemed prudent to convene a group of experts to discuss means of dealing with this potential crisis. The first "solution" offered was to deny the problem. Some people at that time honestly assumed that the polio virus had disappeared from North America and that the lack of vaccination was no threat to the children. Within months of that meeting, however, the first cases of polio in decades appeared. Fortunately they appeared in a wealthy Connecticut community where the vast majority of children had been vaccinated, so the threat of spread was minimal.

These cases forced the health community to consider new approaches to vaccination. It was essential that the Harlem children be protected. Because planning for the future is often a luxury of the wealthy, whereas the poor are preoccupied with daily survival, the health community could not depend on self-enlightened voluntarism. It decided that either a strong incentive—that is, paying parents to bring their children in for vaccination—or a coercive method should be used. The latter, with great reluctance, became the incentive of choice. No children were allowed to enter kindergarten without receiving a polio vaccine, and public schooling is mandatory under penalty of law. This method proved simple and effective. This coercive measure allowed children to grow up with the "freedom" to be unparalyzed at a minimal intrusion on anybody's "autonomy."

To avoid coercion when only coercion will work promotes neither individual freedom nor the common good. To cling to the mythology of pure and rational autonomy even at the cost of children's lives may well be defined as immoral behavior.[12] And what of other unpopular means of influencing behavior short of coercion?

To return to an earlier example: If, like Dr. Elders, we view teenage pregnancy as a yoke that enslaves young girls, are we entitled to encourage these girls to use contraceptives? And what does *encouragement* mean? Should we be permitted to "entice" them into contraceptive usage? And what does *enticement* mean? Should we be permitted to *seduce* them? To *induce* them? To *persuade* them? To *manipulate* them? To *intimidate* them?

Or even to *coerce* them under certain conditions? These often overlapping and sometimes loaded terms demand analysis and understanding.

In a culturally pluralistic society we are obliged to be particularly vigilant and to reexamine principles that were established when our society was more homogeneous. Still, there will always be some legitimate areas for social controls ranging from inducement to coercion: in rearing children; in protecting children; in protecting the helpless; in protecting society and promoting social values, such as beneficence, shared responsibility, and mutual aid; and finally in protecting the environment.

Many contradictions and paradoxes are inherent in our increasingly uncompromising and rigid worship of personal autonomy. Autonomy has become an obstacle to other dimensions of freedom. The emphasis on autonomy has led to a one-sided and self-defeating understanding of freedom. The libertarian crusade to protect everyone's autonomy has led to limits on social policy and social interaction in everyday life that violate common sense and ordinary moral intuitions. So far only health sporadically triumphs over autonomy. We are allowed to prohibit smoking even in open-air arenas, but we are not permitted to control the distribution of automatic weapons.

The growing influence and application of the idea of autonomy is apparent not only in articles and books by political theorists and social philosophers. It permeates the thoughts and feelings, the hopes and concerns, of our whole worldview and way of life. It underlies the growing paranoia, not just of deprived minorities but of the white middle-class, middle-American people who join militias and practice war maneuvers to protect their liberties. A culture of autonomy, in and of itself, is not a sustainable basis for a rich and morally satisfying life of freedom.

American political alignments have not always been as they now are. Deliberate constraints on autonomy and sanctioned uses of coercion were at the heart of the liberal agenda from the New Deal through the Great Society. The mandatory nature of many of our social welfare programs of the past fifty years—now generally accepted as cornerstones of a free society—were all criticized in their day, by conservatives, as unduly coercive. Consider such "erosions of our autonomy" as Social Security, Medicare, and public education.

It is therefore likely that any assault on so revered a concept as autonomy will draw fire from both the right and the left. Nonetheless, we intend to address critically the American understanding of freedom at this crossroads and to offer an analysis of the increasingly libertarian and morally relativistic turn that our culture is taking. To do this, we must examine the wisdom and social effects of the increasing dominance of autonomy as *the* moral imperative in public argument.

The imperialism and arrogance of autonomy must be bridled. Other dimensions of freedom must be recovered and remembered. This work will give us better conceptual tools for principled political argument, for social consensus, and for moral common sense. And it will teach us a much-needed lesson about the proper (that is, morally justified) uses of social controls and coercion in a free society.

In writing this book, we try to adopt the stance of citizens addressing other citizens in a shared space of moral and political community. Many books written today have the explicit intention of waging cultural warfare against ideological enemies. That is not our goal. We are much more concerned with healing a body politic that is fevered by high-pitched rhetoric, beset by antagonistic claims, and in danger of poisoning its own roots and foundations through assault on the very civic and kinship institutions that nourish it. In a quest for diagnosis and healing, conversations among citizens must be first and foremost about fundamental ideas. We intend to demonstrate that personal liberty or autonomy is the linchpin value in America today.

Much that is confusing about social life in America falls into place once we grasp the role of this underlying idea. We ourselves have come to this realization during more than fifteen years of shared work on ethical and social issues in medicine, the life sciences, and public policy. We have often been puzzled and troubled by some of the moral discourse we hear from our fellow citizens, and we have sought to understand what we are hearing, where it is coming from, and how our public discourse could be improved. With these goals in mind, we have tried to write a book that is questioning rather than ideological. That kind of seeking, we believe, is what citizens who ask for the attention and reflection of their fellow citizens should attempt to do.

PART I

the culture
of autonomy

2

A Self of One's Own: The Meaning of Autonomy

> The individual as a type, and individualism as an idea or ideology, are historical developments, social constructs, not fixed and immutable, apart from time and circumstance. The individual is a *creation* of mankind, and it is possible to suggest with fair precision when he first appeared. The moral, psychological, and social attributes of this individual vary sharply from place and moment to place and moment.... The experience of our century both underscores the inadequacies of an absolutist individualism and the dangers of too sweeping an attack upon it.
>
> —IRVING HOWE, *The American Newness: Culture and Politics in the Age of Emerson*

THE PURPOSE OF this book is to understand autonomy and justified coercion from both a philosophical and a psychological standpoint. The three chapters that make up part I, on the culture of autonomy, examine autonomy as a philosophical idea and as an ideal of social and personal life.

This chapter is devoted to a conceptual analysis and a brief intellectual history of the concept of autonomy. It is necessary to begin conceptually and analytically because, we believe, it is important to take the true measure of the culture of autonomy and not to caricature it or to set up a straw man. Only by first appreciating the power of the concept will we be able to comprehend its limitations.

Moral theories are not abstractions invented to keep academic thinkers occupied and to test their ingenuity. Moral ideas initially grow out of the concrete experiences and everyday lives of ordinary people; philosophers

27

then refine these ideas and feed them back into everyday life and experience. Autonomy and its limits are not esoteric matters. How society bal-
ances autonomy and coercion will influence our attitudes and our laws
and social practices on a very wide range of issues, from flag burning to
urinating in the street, from public prayer to the private use of pornography.
What do philosophy and the history of ideas have to tell us about the
assumptions hidden behind such issues?

Defining Autonomy

The word *autonomy* comes from the Greek *autos* (meaning "self") and
nomos (meaning "rule, governance, or law"). Literally, therefore, *autonomy*
means "the state of being self-governed or self-sovereign"; living autonomously means living by a law that you impose on yourself. In other words,
autonomy is the right to live your own life in your own way. The original
usage of the term was political and referred to the self-governing ancient
Greek city-state. Cities had *autonomia* when they made their own laws
and controlled their own affairs, as opposed to being controlled by some
other city or empire.

Over time, particularly in the writings of the eighteenth-century German philosopher Immanuel Kant, the term has also been applied to ethics
and to the individual person. Kant talked mainly about autonomy of the
will or intention; a generation later the English philosopher John Stuart
Mill talked mainly about autonomous action and choice. Both Kant and
Mill have had a tremendous influence on contemporary liberalism.

One widely used college ethics textbook teaches students that autonomy
is the "personal rule of the self that is free from both controlling interference by others and from personal limitations that prevent meaningful
choice. . . . The autonomous individual freely acts in accordance with a
self-chosen plan."[1]

Numerous social and political philosophers express the same general
idea. "To regard himself as autonomous," says Harvard philosopher Thomas
Scanlon, "a person must see himself as sovereign in deciding what to
believe and in weighing competing reasons for action."[2] For his part,
another philosopher, Robert Paul Wolff, places autonomy in the context
of a struggle among human wills for control: "As Kant argued, moral
autonomy is a submission to laws that one has made for oneself. The
autonomous man, insofar as he is autonomous, is not subject to the will

of another. The autonomous . . . man may do what another tells him, but not because he has been told to do it. . . . By accepting as final the commands of the others, he forfeits his autonomy."[3]

Other philosophers and psychologists, such as R. S. Peters and Lawrence Kohlberg, say that autonomy requires a deliberate self-consciousness about obedience to rules. They place it at the pinnacle of moral development. "Children finally pass to the level of autonomy," Peters writes, "when they appreciate that rules are alterable, that they can be criticized and should be accepted or rejected on a basis of reciprocity and fairness. The emergence of rational reflection about rules . . . central to the Kantian conception of autonomy, is the main feature of the final level of moral development."[4] Kohlberg also pictures the best moral agent as standing judgmentally above the existing rules, laws, traditions, habits, and norms of his society, and choosing with rational detachment which rules to follow and which to disregard.[5]

Lawrence Haworth, author of one of the few book-length studies of the concept of autonomy, defines autonomy as having what he calls "critical competence." He writes, "Having critical *competence* a person is first of all active and his activity succeeds in giving effect to his intentions. Having *critical* competence, the active person is sensitive to the results of his own deliberation; his activity is guided by purposes he has thought through and found reasons of his own for pursuing."[6]

These philosophical views of autonomy are widely shared in intellectual circles. Perhaps they are summed up most succinctly, if not most grammatically, by the philosopher Joel Feinberg: "I am autonomous if I rule me, and no one else rules I."[7]

Autonomy is not a single idea but a cluster of closely related, overlapping ideas. Or to put it differently, there are various ways of seeing autonomy, various guises in which it can reveal its moral meaning. Conceptual analysis of the kind we are engaged in here is rather like the meeting of the blind men and the elephant. Each man sees (feels) a different aspect of the beast. Only taken together do these partial perspectives tell us what we want to know.

To grasp what animates the contemporary idea of autonomy, it is important to locate it against the background of the modern worldview that developed in European civilization from roughly the sixteenth century on. The contemporary culture of autonomy in America is derived from this worldview. Drawing on the work of many careful scholars,[8] we sketch the outlines of this worldview and then discuss four distinct but intertwined senses of autonomy that we will later explore in greater detail. They are (1) independence or self-reliance; (2) self-mastery; (3) detachment or irony; and (4) negative liberty.

A HERITAGE OF LIBERATION

The exact historical and intellectual origins of the concept of individual autonomy are difficult to locate. The general ideas that serve as its foundations come from disparate sources and have combined in ways that their authors could not have foreseen and would not approve. Like most of the other ideas central to our culture today, autonomy grew out of the four great transformations that produced the modern world: the Renaissance, the Reformation, the rise of capitalism, and the birth of liberal democracy. All of these build on the special nature of the human being as defined in the biblical tradition, especially the book of Genesis.

The age of cultural and artistic innovation known as the Renaissance contributed to the idea of autonomy by its emphasis on the creative potential and moral significance of the human individual. Received orders and hierarchies, both social and cosmological, had been the framework of medieval thought. But in the fluid and sometimes chaotic social setting of the Italian city-states of the fifteenth and sixteenth centuries, where the Renaissance flourished, individuals of talent, daring, and ambition were able to make their mark. The power of mankind—and by extension the human individual—to create the conditions for its own existence was central to Renaissance humanism and was memorably expressed by Pico della Mirandola in his "Oration on the Dignity of Man." Pico has God say to Adam, "The Nature of all other beings is limited and constrained within the bounds of laws prescribed by Us. Thou, constrained by no limits, in accordance with thine own free will . . . shalt ordain for thyself the limits of thy nature. . . . We have made thee neither of heaven nor of earth . . . so that with freedom of choice and with honor, as though the maker and molder of thyself, thou mayest fashion thyself in whatever shape thou shalt prefer."[9]

The power of the imagery of Genesis sustained the concept of human dignity throughout the Middle Ages. Centuries after Genesis, Macrobius, an influential Latin writer and philosopher, still based his argument for human dignity on the premise that the human race was ennobled by its kinship with the Heavenly Mind, and that of all creatures on earth, only a human shares the mind with heaven and the stars.

The Renaissance and the Reformation helped to expand the notion of human dignity from humankind as a whole to each individual person, and the philosophy of this period also set the stage for later liberalism by stressing the moral importance of the individual as such, apart from any corporate identity or status.[10] Martin Luther, John Calvin, and the other reformers restored a more direct relationship between the individual believer and God by casting aside much of the ritual structure and authoritarian hierarchy that the church had built up over the centuries. Protestantism generally was a more inward-turning form of Christianity than the dominant Catholicism of the time. The faithful would have direct access to God through prayer and to Scripture through translations into the vernacular. The mediation of a learned and authoritative priesthood would no longer be necessary. Individuals had the spiritual capacity in their hearts to receive God's forgiveness, and that, rather than liturgical ceremonies or good works, was the path to salvation.

The reformers, like the humanists who were their contemporaries, also called into question medieval hierarchies and social structures. In this respect the reformers believed that they were returning to the authentic teachings of the early church, especially to the teachings of Saint Paul, who was a key figure in Luther's own theology. One important text from Paul's letter to the Galatians encapsulates this Reformation theme of liberation from the external restraints of law, religious authority, and social division in favor of a new common humanness and inner guidance or direction: "Now before faith came, we were imprisoned and guarded under the law until faith would be revealed. Therefore the law was our disciplinarian until Christ came, so that we might be justified by faith. But now that faith has come, we are no longer subject to a disciplinarian, for in Christ Jesus you are all children of God through faith.[11]

This concept of an "imprisoning law" contrasts sharply with the Jewish view of law as "God's gift" to the people and presages the role Christianity would play in turning away from the communitarian ideal of Judaism and contributing to the newer culture of individualism. Paul himself seemed only too aware of this danger. Recognizing that liberation from the law could unleash a destructive force if misconstrued, he insisted that even

Christian freedom demanded commitment to others, thus preparing the way for an authoritarian church and the Grand Inquisitor: "For you were called to freedom, brothers and sisters; only do not use your freedom as an opportunity for self-indulgence, but through love become slaves to one another. For the whole law is summed up in a single commandment, 'You shall love your neighbor as yourself.' If, however, you bite and devour one another, take care that you are not consumed by one another."[12]

Paul maintained that the need for discipline by the external law (the law given through Moses and the ritual practices of the Jewish people) was past and that justification by faith, or conscience, could take its place. Luther further developed these points extensively in his most important writings (he considered his commentary on Galatians to be his best work) and made them central to his theology. *Sola fide* (justification by faith alone) sums up the entire Reformation.

In a later secular age, after Pauline and Lutheran theology themselves had fallen away, this Protestant appeal to internal conscience rather than external law took Western culture, particularly in predominantly Protestant America, a major step down the road toward a culture of autonomy.

A third historical influence standing behind autonomy is the capitalist economic system and the rise of commercial and entrepreneurial society. The medieval social order was based on an agricultural and military economy, and its values were openly hostile to the notions of private property, social mobility, interest, profits, and investment. The new urban-based commercial society of capitalism introduced precisely these values into European life in the early modern period. Capitalism was a way of life that forced individuals to break out of traditional roles, obligations, and expectations. It rewarded risk taking and innovation. Combined with Protestant individualism in various ways, capitalism was the cradle of autonomy's notions of independence, self-reliance, and working for self-satisfaction and fulfillment, as the German sociologist Max Weber demonstrated in *The Protestant Ethic and the Spirit of Capitalism*.[13]

Finally, autonomy was born in the political revolutions of the seventeenth and eighteenth centuries that overthrew the rule of absolutist monarchies in England (1642 and 1688), the American colonies (1776), and France (1789), and replaced them with regimes whose claim to authority and legitimacy was based on the notion of consent of the governed. The intellectual basis for these new revolutionary regimes was the political theory of natural rights and the social contract, most powerfully developed by thinkers like Thomas Hobbes, John Locke, and Jean-Jacques Rousseau. They taught modern society to believe that the state or political society exists in order to protect the rights and serve the interests of the individuals who make it up; individuals do not exist to serve the interests of the state. From this theory has come not only the ideal of autonomy but the whole political framework that we call liberal democracy and liberalism.

Rooted in humanism, Protestantism, capitalism, and natural rights theory, liberalism has been the American political philosophy par excellence. We have virtually no other. In its historical sense, "liberalism"—so unfashionable these days—encompasses the entire ideological spectrum of American politics today, from those who favor a large regulatory and economic role for government, whom we call liberals, to those who emphasize market competition and voluntary organizations, whom we call conservatives and libertarians.

In all of its American guises, liberalism has always been the guardian of the individual against the state and against any established church. However, liberalism has not only been concerned with state power and authority. Over time, as liberal political philosophy has developed and the notion of autonomy has been refined, mistrust of the state has broadened to become a more generalized mistrust of society and culture as a whole. As liberals have recognized, society and culture themselves impose limits on autonomy in the form of moral norms and mores, which may be as powerfully and coercively enforced in informal social settings as any formal law is by the government. Liberalism worries about the tyranny of the majority and the tyranny of public opinion as much as it worries about the tyranny of the state.

Thus embedded in the liberal tradition are several important tenets that give autonomy its extraordinary moral power and appeal. They can be summarized as follows. One tenet is *moral individualism*, the belief that the human individual is the center of the moral universe, the subject of ultimate worth to whose well-being all other things that may be said to have moral value must finally contribute. Another is the remarkable notion, so beautifully expressed by Pico, that *man makes himself*; that the basic features of society are ultimately products of human choice and artifice, and as such the social world is a human world, a world fashioned not by God or nature but by the amazingly plastic, adaptive human will. Perhaps deliberately echoing Pico, but at any rate certainly expressing a thoroughly humanistic theme, poet Archibald MacLeish stated Americans' own home-grown version of this idea in his 1943 lecture, "Unimagined America": "We have, and we know we have, the abundant means to bring our boldest dreams to pass—to create for ourselves whatever world we have the courage to desire. We have the metal and the men to take this country down, if we please to take it down, and to build it again as we please to build it . . . to brighten the air, to clean the wind, to live as men in this Republic, free men, should be living."[14]

The final root idea underlying autonomy is the doctrine of *moral choice or consent*. The moral life of the individual is made up of relationships, commitments, and obligations that the individual has freely chosen, not those into which she was born or that were imposed upon her. Rather, autonomy means living in accordance with rules that one gives to oneself. If an autonomous person does her duty, it is because she has freely and rationally chosen to do so. Autonomy gives us no way of understanding duty—or moral responsibility—outside the domain of rational choice or will. This places a burden on reason that it cannot sustain. In this burden lies both the glory and the Achilles's heel of autonomy.

AUTONOMY AS INDEPENDENCE

Human beings are born biologically premature, so that unlike most mammals, many of our neurological and physical functions and all of our behavioral capacities exist at birth in potential form only. To come to fruition, these potentials must be molded by a social environment. Newborn colts can stand within a few minutes after birth and run within hours. They carry practically the entire behavioral repertoire of adult horses with them from the first. Humans, however, are born incomplete and remain dependent for an exceptionally long time. Our behavioral repertoire gradually grows, develops, and becomes much more complex, as does our conscious awareness. Maturation, socialization, just plain growing up—call it what you will—involves a movement from dependence and incompleteness to greater independence and maturation.

These biological and psychological facts of human nature are the conditions that make autonomy possible in the first place, although by no means do they guarantee actually achieving it. This universal experience of our species—this journey from dependence to independence—is the matrix from which our autonomy crystallizes; it is in the social environment of dependence that we build an autonomous adult sense of an independent self.

Independence and self-reliance are crucial aspects of autonomy that lend it great emotional force and moral appeal. Autonomy suggests that persons are able to stand upright on their own two legs; they can go their own way, walk their own path, and take a stand. This is a mark of human self-realization. It is the path we were meant to travel. To be dependent is to remain incomplete, unfulfilled. Moreover, to be dependent is to be held back, to be confined and constrained to conform, when one instead should move away, stretch one's own limbs, and find one's own shape.

Ralph Waldo Emerson is America's great teacher of autonomy as independence. In his essay "Self-Reliance," he declared that "Society everywhere is in conspiracy against the manhood of every one of its members. . . . Society is a joint-stock company, in which the members agree, for the better securing of his bread to each shareholder, to surrender the liberty and culture of the eater. The virtue in most request is conformity. Self-reliance is its aversion. . . . Whoso would be a man must be a nonconformist."[15]

AUTONOMY AS SELF-MASTERY

Autonomy is more than self-sufficiency; it is self-sufficiency with intelligence and purpose. There is a difference between no one being in charge of you (*anomia*) and being in charge of yourself (*autonomia*). Autonomy is sometimes used to mean one and sometimes the other. It would probably be clearer to use the term *anomie* to refer to the former, and reserve *autonomy* for the latter, but our everyday language will never be this precise.

When autonomy as self-mastery is invoked, metaphors of private property are never far away, just as independence draws on metaphors of maturation and liberty draws on metaphors of space. To be master of yourself is to belong to yourself.

A powerful expression of autonomy as self-mastery is explored in Toni Morrison's novel *Beloved*. Morrison writes of the experience of freedom first sensed by Baby Suggs—matriarch of the family whose deeply scarred life the novel examines. Baby Suggs's slave son, Halle, purchases her freedom from a sympathetic master, and she crosses the river from Sweet Home plantation in Kentucky into southern Ohio and freedom:

When Mr. Garner agreed to the arrangements with Halle, and when Halle looked like it meant more to him that she go free than anything in the world, she let herself be taken 'cross the river . . . when she stepped foot on free ground she . . . knew that there was nothing like it in this world . . . suddenly she saw her hands and thought with a clarity as simple as it was dazzling, "These hands belong to me. These *my* hands." Next she felt a knocking in her chest and discovered something else new: her own heartbeat. Had it been there all along?[16]

Autonomy as self-mastery has taken up permanent residence in our modern moral imagination. Once you have crossed with Baby Suggs to the north bank of the Ohio, there is no turning back.

Moreover, if we cannot turn back, we also cannot—or should not—understate what the idea of self-mastery implies. Some theorists of autonomy, such as John Rawls and Ronald Dworkin, hold that autonomy is "neutral" with respect to any particular substantive conception of the human good.[17] What they mean by this is that autonomy has no inside; it is an empty freedom waiting to be filled with choices, like a house to be filled with furniture, or a garden with flowers and shrubs. Neutral autonomy also has no direction, no purpose beyond itself. It is the freedom to choose and the activity of choosing that matter, not what is chosen. This makes autonomy like the expensive treadmills so many Americans buy today to go nowhere in particular, but just to go. Autonomy, here, is nothing but a bulky piece of equipment if it is not used. Many Americans think of autonomy as choice for its own sake.

We believe that as a philosophical understanding of the meaning and value of autonomy, this conception is inadequate in two different ways. Self-mastery means something more than "do your own thing." Baby Suggs knew this. What she received when she crossed the Ohio River was not merely the chance, as the U.S. Army recruiting slogan says, to "be all that you can be." As an unblinking observer of being black in America, Toni Morrison has no time, and less patience, for such notions. Arriving on the "free" soil of southern Ohio in the days before the Civil War, Baby Suggs had no equality and precious little opportunity, and she was far too old and tired to be filling up empty jugs of autonomy with her lifestyle choices.

The experience Morrison is talking about when Baby Suggs discovers self-mastery is not something Baby Suggs has to fill; it is something that fills her. It transforms and recreates her anew, paradoxically by letting her discover a self that was there all along—obscured by the weight of slavery, which is not only a set of laws, practices, and power relationships but also a prison house of images, symbols, defenses, and deceptions. Ideas matter. The poet William Blake called ideas such as slavery "mind-forg'd manacles."[18] It is a necessary good for a human being to rise above them so that you can see yourself plain and be yourself truly.

This is not all Morrison has to teach us about the subject of freedom. *Beloved* goes on to explore a different form of self-possession and self-mastery that is compatible with human interdependence and life in a community of mutual aid and reciprocal obligation.

After Baby Suggs goes to Ohio, her daughter-in-law, Sethe, runs away from Sweet Home plantation with her children in order to join Baby Suggs. In the following passage Sethe describes her flight and her experience of freedom:

> I did it. I got us all out. Without Halle too. Up till then it was the only thing I ever did on my own. I birthed them and I got em out and it wasn't no accident. I did that. Me having to look out. Me using my own head. But it was more than that. It was a kind of selfishness I never knew nothing about before. It felt good. Good and right. I was big . . . and deep and wide and when I stretched out my arms all my children could get in between. I was *that* wide. Look like I loved em more after I got here. Or maybe I couldn't love em proper in Kentucky because they wasn't mine to love.[19]

Being free enables Sethe to love her children "proper." It also enables the African American people in the Ohio town to form a community of care, concern, and love. They are able to care for one another because they are free. When they were slaves, of course, they could help one another, tend one another, have all the universal human emotions of sympathy, compassion, tenderness, and love. But they could not engage in the structured activity of caring and responding *as a community* because the mind-forged, law-forged, and whip-forged manacles of slavery deprived them of the circumstances necessary to make their own community. Freedom makes community possible. But taking care of each other, being a person in the fabric of such a community, is what gives freedom its point.

Freedom and commitment, independence and dependence, rights and restraints—these are not, in the final reckoning, contraries.

It is interesting and apt that Morrison should choose the word *selfishness* here and use it without, insofar as we can detect, the slightest negative moral connotation. It is not the selfishness of taking or grasping to which she refers; it is the capacity to embrace and draw in. Ordinary garden-variety selfishness makes one small; this experience of freedom made Sethe big, as big and deep and wide as Christ on the Cross: "when I stretched out my arms all my children could get in between."

AUTONOMY AS IRONY

Closely related to the idea of self-mastery is that sense of autonomy you experience when you exercise socially detached, rational judgment in the circumstances of your life. Autonomy calls for a hyperconsciousness about the social rules you obey, the roles you play, and even the type of person you are. This does not mean that you have to stop obeying rules or stop playing roles; it does suggest that you should obey only those rules and play only those roles that have passed rational and moral muster by your autonomous, judging ego. Kant made autonomy in this sense the essence of ethics. His major successors in nineteenth-century philosophy—Hegel, Kierkegaard, and Nietzsche—found Kant's thought profoundly flawed; but they all understood only too well the significance of what he had discovered in modern man. They called this sense of autonomy the "unhappy" or "ironic" consciousness.

Ironic autonomy is restless, unsatisfied, and disruptive; and it is supposed to be. One of the best literary studies of it is Molière's play *The Misanthrope*. Alceste, the title character, is a man who refuses to put up with hypocrisy, social convention, and the inauthenticity of a highly stylized and precious aristocratic society. When his suave friend Philinte tells him that his frankness and endless criticism of social customs has put people off, Alceste replies:

So much the better; just what I wish to hear,
No news could be more grateful to my ear.
All men are so detestable in my eyes
I should be sorry if they thought me wise.

Later he adds: "My God! It chills my heart to see the ways / Men come to terms with evil nowadays."

Philinte nonetheless continues to press his friend to take a different posture toward the world:

This world requires a pliant rectitude
Too stern a virtue makes one stiff and rude,
Good sense views all extremes with detestation,
And bids us to be noble in moderation.
The rigid virtues of the ancient days . . .
Ask of us too lofty a perfection.[20]

Molière, whose own sympathies lay with the worldly wisdom of Philinte, treats Alceste's moralism harshly as the play goes on. The misanthrope is revealed and ridiculed as a self-absorbed and insensitive prig rather than the courageous and virtuous character he claims to be.

Perhaps Molière is right, and Alceste's own self-deception does give the lie to his explicit criticism of everyone else's pretense. However, today we are closer to Alceste's spirit of uncompromising personal integrity than to the playwright's "pliant rectitude." The refined manners and elaborate social ritual of the French aristocracy have become museum pieces, whereas the cultural type of the authentic and autonomous self has flourished.

Habit, ritual behavior, and automatic response would seem inappropriate to that self, a betrayal of one's gift of autonomy. We, on the other hand, argue that these emotion-based and socially embedded aspects of behavior are essential and should not be sharply pitted against reason and reasonableness. Although the capacity for rational judgment is often important, much of human behavior (much more than we like to admit) is nonrationally determined. For now, it is sufficient to realize that this sense of autonomy, illusion though it may be, is deeply rooted in our culture. Its power and appeal for modern Americans are best appreciated by recalling that it has its roots in the political realm and in the revolutionary legacy of the past three hundred years that produced the Western liberal democracies.

The political theories that guided the English, American, and French revolutions imagined that once there had been—and that there could he created again—an explicit social contract in which each person is asked to detach himself from all traditions, habits, beliefs, and allegiances, and then to decide what political and social institutions to build from the ground up. This is, at least to some extent, what the American Founders were doing at the Constitutional Convention in 1787, when they scrapped the Articles of Confederation and wrote a different governmental structure into the new constitution. What's more, they saw this as their obligation and privilege. They were autonomous men.

Few of us, fortunately, are ever faced with such a founding moment, for surely we would make a mess of it. But the style of moral thinking introduced by social contract theory—from Thomas Hobbes and John Locke in the seventeenth century to John Rawls and many others today—continues to be used every day to provide a workable test for political and ethical legitimacy. When faced with a rule or a policy that you have moral questions about, this aspect of autonomy does not tell you to ask how much happiness in general the rule would produce, or whether it would promote your own selfish interest, or whether it is compatible with God's commands. Instead you are to ask if rational, detached persons would consent to this rule or policy if they were judging it. If something cannot stand up to ironic rational scrutiny, consign it to the flames.

AUTONOMY AS NEGATIVE LIBERTY

The richest sense of autonomy and probably the most important one in America today is the notion of autonomy as negative liberty. To understand how autonomy and liberty (or freedom) are related, a good starting point is the distinction between negative and positive liberty that was first suggested by the British political theorist Sir Isaiah Berlin in his important essay "Two Concepts of Liberty."

Negative liberty has to do with establishing a zone of privacy and noninterference around each person, a zone within which the person can exercise his own faculties and pursue his own life in his own way. Berlin explains that "The defense of liberty consists in the 'negative' goal of warding off interference. To threaten a man with persecution unless he submits to a life in which he exercises no choices of his goals; to block before him every door but one, no matter how noble the prospect upon which it opens, or how benevolent the motives of those who arrange this, is to sin against the truth that he is a man, a being with a life of his own to live."[21]

Autonomy understood as negative liberty appeals to metaphors of space. It wants elbowroom—a place of one's own. It is the single-family dwelling of ethics. Negative liberty requires fences and boundaries for protection against outside intruders. It rests on a conflict-ridden and antagonistic picture of social existence, in which each individual struggles with everyone else to control his own patch of ground. Negative liberty does not appeal to Napoleons or Don Juans. It appeals to ordinary folks who simply wish not to be dominated, who wish to be left alone.

The rights most closely linked to this sense of autonomy are those classic political or civil rights that protect the individual from the power of the state, as enshrined in the Bill of Rights in the U.S. Constitution: freedom of speech, assembly, and religion; freedom from unreasonable search and seizure; security of home and property. These ideas were the basis of Justice Louis Brandeis's elevation of "the right to be let alone"[22] as the transcendent right.

This traditional liberal idea of securing for the individual freedom from the power of the state has been extended by the civil rights revolution to include security from the interference of other people in private or social life. More recently, in the era of no-fault divorce, it has been extended to family life. But is the relationship of the powerful state to the helpless individual a model we wish to assume for all relationships among people? When someone has a right to negative liberty, it means that others have a corresponding obligation not to trespass, not to intrude uninvited upon the person's zone of privacy and self-determination. We surely cannot oblige parents not to intrude upon the privacy of their children. The parent who acts toward a child as we would have the state act toward the individual would be a negligent parent.

Autonomy is also linked to liberty in another sense, through what Berlin and others have called *positive liberty*. Positive liberty is very close to self-mastery and detached judgment. Berlin explicates it this way:

The "positive" sense of the word "liberty" derives from the wish on the part of the individual to be his own master. I wish my life and decisions to depend on myself, not on external forces of whatever kind. I wish to be the instrument of my own, not of other men's, acts of will. I wish to be a subject, not an object; to be moved by reasons, by conscious purposes, which are my own, not by causes which affect me, as it were, from outside. I wish to be somebody, not nobody; a doer—deciding, not being decided for, self-directed and not acted upon by external nature or by other men as if I were a thing, or an animal, or a slave incapable of playing a human role, that is, of conceiving goals and policies of my own and realizing them.[23]

One is free in the positive sense when one's reason, one's higher self, is in charge of one's conduct. Negative liberty is the absence of control by others; positive liberty is more like self-control. Autonomy as positive liberty rests on the insight that human self-sufficiency is limited and that freedom often requires the assistance of others. This insight has led to an expansion of the concept of rights into what has been called *positive rights*.

Rights are moral (or legal) claims that a person makes against one or more other people to protect or promote his or her freedom. Whereas the Bill of Rights lists essentially negative rights, detailing what the state cannot do to us, positive rights are what the state owes us. Positive rights are sometimes called "welfare rights" or "social rights." Public education, income maintenance programs such as Social Security and Aid to Families with Dependent Children, food stamps, disability benefits, unemployment compensation, health care for the elderly (Medicare) and the poor (Medicaid), and handicapped access to public spaces are forms of assistance that have been deemed positive rights.

Since the time of the New Deal in the United States, and well back into the late nineteenth century in England and the western European countries, arguments have arisen between so-called liberals and conservatives about the scope and justification of welfare programs of this kind. The usual way of explaining these debates is to say that liberals and conservatives share the same basic end—namely, the protection and promotion of autonomy—but disagree about the best means to achieve that end. Conservatives believe that private market competition will provide the necessary conditions for individuals to enjoy the freedom to pursue their ends. Liberals believe that active government programs and regulation are necessary because the private market will fail to help those most disadvantaged and in need of assistance.

There is a more enlightening way to understand the central political arguments surrounding the liberal welfare state. Welfare state arguments are in fact the expression of clashes between negative liberty and positive liberty. Although debates like the recent one over health care reform pit government regulation against market competition, that is a false opposition and an illusory choice. In modern capitalism it is unlikely that markets could function without some government regulation and the infusion of public funds to stimulate economic growth; similarly, governments would collapse in fiscal and political crisis were it not for the economic prosperity and employment created by corporate and small business competition.

What is actually at stake in these debates is the emphasis given to different aspects of autonomy. Negative and positive rights and liberties clash. When I ask to be left alone, it would seem to be an easy request for others to fulfill, but not if they need my help to enjoy their freedom to realize their goals. Does a physician have a "right to be let alone" to pursue his golf game in the presence of a hemorrhaging player who is blocking his way? That specific issue had to be hammered out in the courts of law.

Positive obligations—obligations of active assistance instead of negative forbearance—impinge on negative liberty. When a conflict arises, which is to have moral priority: an individual's claims to privacy, security, and noninterference, or someone else's claim to be assisted so that he can fulfill his life goals?

American women have a negative right not to be interfered with by the government (or by anybody else) if they want to have an early abortion. American law, and at least the liberal part of American morality, both affirm this right; they say it is her body, her choice, her autonomy. However, that same woman does not have a right to have a particular doctor help her with an abortion. If any particular doctor does not want to do abortions because he finds them morally objectionable, he does not have to. That is autonomy too. What would happen if none of the doctors in the country were willing to perform abortions? A woman's negative right not to be hindered from having an abortion would have to become a positive right to be helped in having one. Not hindering is different from helping. Would we then have to force doctors to perform abortions even though they would rather not? How would we do it? Through financial incentives? Conscription into the army, where physicians follow orders, as we threatened to do with striking workers in essential industries during World War II? Thus far we have been fortunate that enough doctors agree with a woman's right to choose, so the dilemma has not come to a head. However, the number of doctors who perform abortions is dwindling, and most obstetrics training programs today no longer teach young physicians how to do the procedure.

The world of autonomy as negative liberty is a world of absences and omissions. As such, it is a clean well-lighted place. One of autonomy's best emblems is the revolutionary-era flag that shows a coiled snake and the motto "Don't Tread on Me." The world of positive liberty is a messier space, filled with shadows. It is a much more human space. In it, people do things to and with one another. They cannot get by simply by steering clear. "Don't tread on me" gives way to "Help me up." In an interactive world, influence, social control, and even coercion are not the enemies of autonomy; they define an environment necessary for the nourishing of freedom. Autonomy understood as positive liberty requires rules, defined roles, relationships, and duties of commission, not merely omission.

What Do We Have to Lose?

In order, to illuminate the special role of autonomy in our culture, Joel Feinberg, one of the leading theorists of autonomy, has asked what would be missing if we lived in a society that did not understand the concepts of autonomy and rights. He imagined a prosperous and benevolent society, not tyranny or despotism. He imagined a society in which individuals possessed all the other virtues and lived by the Ten Commandments and the Golden Rule. Even in such a good and happy society, Feinberg said, something essential to morality and humanity would be lacking. Individuals would not be able to make claims on each other for dignity and respect.

Autonomy allows one person to demand respect from another as a matter of right. Not to ask meekly for respect as a matter of goodwill, friendship, or charity, but to *demand* it. Proudly. And not necessarily because of some accomplishment, but just because one is a person, an adult human being, a first-class member of the moral community. It is through the concepts of autonomy and rights that we gain our sense of identity as moral persons and free agents worthy of the respect of others.[24]

The ideal of autonomy releases tremendous moral energy by allowing human beings to feel secure in their own moral worth. The terrible enervation experienced by the once-vital societies of Central Europe during the years of communist rule is proof enough of what happens when people, having once tasted autonomy in their lives, suffer it to be extinguished.

Cultural and social structures such as norms, laws, and institutions are empty and desiccated without the restless, dynamic energy that autonomy unleashes.

In communist societies democracy was the official constitution, and all the politically correct laws and rights were on the books. However, the gulf between theory and reality was so glaring that no one took the official ideals seriously—least of all the party leaders. Cynicism took the place of a sense of moral self-worth and dignity. Under these conditions, social and cultural goods are dissipated, and passion is drained from everyday life. The desire and aspiration that keep societies vital are heightened by autonomy, by the sense that one belongs to oneself.

In addition to preserving this vitality, autonomy serves society by challenging conventions and accepted ways of life. It is a catalyst for moral growth and social enlightenment. Psychologists like Kohlberg and Peters see autonomy as a sign of moral adulthood in the individual; only autonomous persons are truly grown-up, regardless of their age.

Change is always frightening. Circumstances, people, or beliefs that provoke change are therefore liable to be suppressed. Respecting individual autonomy and rights is one of the ways a society has to curb its own resistance to change and to protect nonconformity as an agent of change in its midst.

Autonomy does not come without costs. It tolerates the freedom of the unlovable and disreputable, as well as the freedom of the respectable advanced thinker. To respect autonomy only when it is cost-free or not socially disruptive is to fail to take it seriously. It is often most valuable when it is most dangerous, most despised. Precisely the point of individual rights, after all, is that they must be preserved when they are threatened.

The rights protecting individual autonomy are not particularly important, or even essential, when people are exercising behavior that is universally accepted. These rights are not even all that important in a climate of toleration, where people are prepared to defer even to those of whom they do not really approve. The rights protecting autonomy do become very important, however, when some people detest what others are doing, when they have "good reasons"—especially moral or religious ones—to oppose or forbid that which others would say or do. In our times, the central moral role of holding that banner aloft has been performed by the American Civil Liberties Union (ACLU).

Galileo was a dangerous man to the arbiters of morality in his day. We must learn to live with such dangerous men. At their inception, the various philosophical, religious, and political traditions that have forged our modern culture of autonomy were viewed as dissenting and heterodox. We ought to have learned from our own historical experience that those behaviors that seem most objectionable and most natural to suppress are the ones that need protecting the most. They will often guide the way to tomorrow's truth.

What about the deviant behavior that is only too evident in modern life? How do we protect the eccentric from the pressures of social conformity, without at the same time turning our backs on self-destructive behavior that may in actuality be a tacit plea for help? In what direction should we err—toward too little interference or too much? With the expression of political ideas we should, of course, err in the direction of toleration. But nonpolitical statements of lifestyle must not be conflated with political freedom. When our moral common sense is eclipsed by rigid protections of negative liberty, terrible mistakes can be made.

Remember the fate of William Black, whose story we told at the beginning of chapter 1. America didn't tread on William Black, it stepped over him. Seemingly mindless autonomy-respecting policies, like the one followed by the EMS workers that day, do not come from nowhere. They are responses to real abuses of individual rights and liberties in the past. But we must find some balance, some middle ground. Our society must be both free and decent; it must behave itself, standing somewhere between the political abuse of psychiatry in the Soviet gulag (or the abuses of involuntary commitment in some American psychiatric hospitals) and a hands-off autonomy. William Black should not have been allowed to die of "autonomy"—not in the silent shadow of Saint Luke the Physician.

3

Land of the Free: Autonomy in American Life Today

If I am not for myself, who is for me?
—HILLEL, Babylonian Talmud, *Aboth* I:14

THUS FAR WE have tried to convey the meaning of autonomy through philosophical definitions and an account of its nuanced history in the Western intellectual and political tradition. We turn now to the place of autonomy in the climate of ideas in America today.

Our aim is to provide a sense of how the notion of autonomy has embedded itself in everyday thinking and feeling. The point is not that people always use the word *autonomy* to describe what they are claiming, thinking, and longing for. A host of words make up the vocabulary of personal aspiration in the United States today: the good life, security, rights, privacy, peace of mind, steady work, respect, fairness, equal treatment, decency, an even break. What links these diverse hopes and values is an underlying notion of personal liberty, self-expression, self-reliance, and noninterference. What makes the concept of autonomy so ubiquitous—and what makes it meaningful for us to speak about a culture of autonomy—is the fact that a peculiarly individualistic interpretation is placed on nearly every social and moral value in American life today.

Through thirty years of jurisprudence and legislation that has weakened state authority and strengthened individual rights, privacy, and entitlements, autonomy has bored deeply into the laws of the land.[1] Nothing inherent in civil rights laws, for example, requires that they be interpreted in individualistic terms; their meaning could easily be construed in terms of nondiscrimination or equality. But such is the gravitational force of autonomy in our way of life that in America today civil rights have become more a framework for individual claims against others than a framework for social solidarity; they are more about demanding positions that have been previously denied than about building a moral community of equal citizens. At times such a confrontational interpretation of moral and legal rights may be necessary to get the attention of the powerful and to bring about social change. If these tactics take on a life of their own, however, movements for social reform can easily lose their moral vision and original sense of purpose.

The tendency to cut all social values from the cloth of autonomy has been vaguely felt more than carefully analyzed; it is taken for granted, like a familiar but uniform landscape, but not critically assessed. Our intention here is first to call attention to a moral sensibility that views social issues and values through the lens of autonomy, and second to call that lens into question. It is a powerful lens, not one to be lightly or simply dismissed. (The true measure of autonomy in American life will not be taken merely by pointing out instances of its "abuse.") But it is also a distorting lens, particularly when we allow it to magnify the individual out of all background, context, and proportion.

Everyday Autonomy

Like so many English words that derive from ancient Greek or Latin, *autonomy* has a somewhat precious air about it. Philosophers are obsessed with it, whereas many ordinary people manage their daily lives without much reference to it. It is a word more at home in a classroom, a courtroom, or a congressional hearing than on a talk-radio program, around a suburban dinner table, or over open lunchboxes at a construction site. It is therefore easy to underestimate its importance in Americans' day-to-day existence. Although the word autonomy is not often used in everyday conversation, the *idea* it stands for is everywhere. Americans live, breathe, and dream autonomy. It is our benchmark of success in life; it is what we reward and admire in others and strive for in ourselves.

The United States features history's longest-running democratic experiment, now well into its third century, and our greatest achievement so far has been not peace or even material prosperity but the unprecedented measure of freedom and autonomy we grant to individuals in their lives. The autonomy of the individual represents America's greatest moral strength and now, peculiarly, its most insidious moral danger. The arrival of terrorism in the United States on September 11, 2001, has led many to pose this very issue, but often in a quite simplistic way. Lax security at airports and other public places, the ability to smuggle weapons, bombs, or foreign operatives into the country, legal limits on law enforcement agencies in terms of surveillance and privacy protections—these and other problems have been taken as symptomatic of the inherent vulnerability of a free and open society. No doubt individuals will have to put up with more delays and restrictions in the future. More seriously, some individuals will be singled out for discriminatory treatment on the basis of fear, prejudice, and guilt by association. Again, that may be an unavoidable price some will pay for the sake of greater security and peace of mind of others. Yet, as troubling as threats of this violent and murderous kind are, the more slow acting, invisible threats that tend to undermine our core institutions and values are—or should be—more troubling still.

Autonomy's stock is on the rise with ordinary people, not just academic intellectuals. It has been elevated to first place among the things we value and want to protect. The various human and civil rights movements prominent since the 1960s have accelerated this trend: civil rights for racial minorities, women's rights, abortion rights, gay rights, consumer rights, even patients' rights and the right to die. Along with these rights movements has come a distrust of all authority. *Paternalism*—making people do what is good for them even if they do not want to do it—is certainly out of favor, in some areas rightly so. People mistrust paternalistic professionals like doctors and other experts, and large majorities of middle-class voters now claim to want paternalistic government "off their backs."

In this era of distrust and litigation, when children have brought suits for "divorce" from their parents, it may not be long before even parents won't be able to get away with paternalism. Beyond a certain point, however, disrespect for authority destroys the trust essential to communal living. It will eventually undermine the very cultural and institutional infrastructure upon which rights, liberties, and personal autonomy themselves depend.

In dealings between professionals and clients, a conscious concern for autonomy has led clients to demand a much more active and controlling role. Nowhere is this more evident than in the practice of medicine, where an ethical and legal emphasis on the patient's right of "informed consent" has supplanted the days of benevolent physician paternalism.

It is easy to see the ways in which this represents a gain; individuals are better protected from the exploitation inherent in the unequal power of the professional-client relationship. It is less easy, but no less important, to see what has been lost. Professional beneficence and dedication to the well-being of the client has suffered considerably from the recent autonomy-oriented and adversarial atmosphere. This loss is particularly apparent in medicine, where informed consent—the patient's right to know the diagnosis and to decide upon treatment options—now reigns supreme. Today it is in fact the leading principle underlying modern medical ethics in this country, although not in others. In more homogeneous Sweden, where trust between physician and patients was a given, informed consent has had little sway until very recent times.

Truth-telling is at the heart of consent, and a physician's moral concern for the relationship with the patient ought to surround and inform that truth-telling. But in some cases that concern has given way to a rigid moral formalism, reinforced by fear of malpractice liability. In a word, truth-telling has sometimes now become "truth-dumping"—candor with a vengeance. Information is given with little or no attention to the context—intellectual, emotional, and social—within which that information will be received and understood. In the past, it was part of medical ethics, and part of the professional experience of most physicians, to agonizingly weigh how much information the patient should be given in the name of truth and the right to know, on the one hand, against how much pain, anxiety, and family dislocation the patient should be shielded from, on the other. Increasingly, that traditional dilemma no longer concerns physicians, as communication takes on an increasingly routinized, bureaucratic, and impersonal quality.

In other social contexts, many powerful movements on the right wing of the ideological spectrum have further reinforced the culture of autonomy. Economic conservatives extol the virtues of free market competition; philosophical libertarians defend private property rights and resist government taxes; and most uncompromising of all, militant anarchists, such as the citizen militia groups, seem to reject any form of governmental or social authority. Although these latter-day anarchists upset and offend liberal defenders of autonomy, it is impossible to deny that the value the liberal community places on personal autonomy is one powerful motivating factor behind the antigovernment mood sweeping the country at the grassroots level today. The right-wing militias are simply the most extreme manifestation of that mood.

In a thoughtful article on the ideology and ethos of right-wing militia groups, Denis Johnson relates his own fascination with the independence and self-reliance these groups both symbolize and idolize. Having become acquainted with members of these militia groups in Alaska, Johnson was invited to spend his honeymoon at a remote site in the Bonanza Hills southwest of Anchorage. Johnson's description of his experience is a good example of the grass-roots level meaning of autonomy:

> My wife and I honeymooned that month at David's mining operation in the Bonanza Hills. A plane dropped us off . . . [and] Cindy and I lived without any contact with what I had up to then believed to be the world, in a place without human community, authority, or law, seventy miles from the nearest person. . . . Things I'd never thought about became uppermost: matches and tools and, above all, clarity of thought and the ability to improvise. We had to stay focused in our senses, ever mindful of our tasks, because what we'd brought and who we were was all we had. At last, whatever happened to us could only be *our* fault or bad fortune, and fixing it *our* responsibility. We realized our lives had never before been our own—*our* lives. I had always lived under the protection of what I've since heard called "The Nanny State": Big Mom, ready to patch me up, bail me out, calm me down, and only a three-digit phone call away. Just the same, it's a free country. I'd always taken for granted that the government looked after the basics and left me free to enjoy my liberty. Now I wasn't so sure. This little taste of real autonomy excited in me a craving for it. Maybe I wanted freedom from the government's care and protection. Maybe I wanted freedom from any government at all. I felt grateful for people like David, who'd run away from home and could get along for weeks at a time in a place like the Bonanza Hills.[2]

The value Americans place on autonomy is not new, of course. Marching to one's own drummer has been the thing to do in the United States since well before there was a United States. The Pilgrims who landed at Plymouth Rock in 1620 were only the first in a long line of immigrants who came to the New World seeking the liberty to live their lives in their own way. Although autonomy has been around for a long time, it has never been the only value; it has always coexisted with other values, and with other ideas about what constitutes the good life. Even in the revolutionary period, some shrewd observers of Americans' fierce sense of independence and love of liberty warned that freedom alone cannot sustain the entire social fabric upon which freedom itself is based.

The historian Gordon Wood found this concern expressed by one Samuel Mitchill of New York in 1800, who complained that everyone in America wanted independence: "First independence from Great Britain, then independence of the states from each other, then independence of the people from the government, and 'lastly, the members of society be equally independent of each other.' "[3]

The conditions of extreme individualism that were already a reality on the American frontier (which then meant Buffalo, not the Bonanza Hills) were also an inherent cultural impulse faced by the entire society. At the heart of America, Mitchill thought, lay a self-defeating condition in which there would be "no private or publick associations for common good, every Man standing single," and where "every man is for himself alone and has no regard for any person farther than he can make him subservient to his own views."

Reflecting on the alarm felt by people like Mitchill, Wood observes that "authority of every sort seemed unable to resist these endless challenges. By what right did authority claim obedience? was the question being asked of every institution, every organization, every individual. It was as if the Revolution had set in motion a disintegrative force that could not be stopped."[4]

The very essence of the Constitution and the Bill of Rights, according to that distinguished defender of the individual, Justice Louis Brandeis, rests in our private right to run our own lives. In 1928 he wrote that "They [the makers of the Constitution] conferred, as against the government, the right to be let alone—the most comprehensive of rights and the right most valued by civilized men."[5]

This was an idea before its time. The Great Depression and the New Deal of Franklin Roosevelt ushered in a period of governmental paternalism, beneficence, and community consciousness that persisted through World War II. In the Depression people were not insisting that the government leave them alone, they were asking the government to take care of them—

to provide them with food, shelter, and work. And the government did. During the war years the individual repaid that government by sacrificing self-interest for service to his country and its ideals.

During the past thirty years America has undergone yet another shift in emphasis, this time away from social values and toward individualistic values. Autonomy has ceased to be one value among many and has assumed pride of place as the moral touchstone of our personal lives and our social institutions. Even as our laws have been changed to grant individuals ever wider latitude for freedom of choice and self-expression (the so-called "rights revolution"), our culture ranks autonomy first among ethical values. Yale legal philosopher Bruce Ackerman expresses this shift vividly: "A respect for the autonomy of persons is one of the . . . main highways to the liberal state. . . . It is . . . not necessary for autonomy to be the only good thing; it suffices for it to be the best thing that there is."[6]

Autonomy now preempts civility, altruism, paternalism, beneficence, community, mutual aid, and other moral values that essentially tell a person to set aside his own interests in favor of the interests of other people or the good of something larger than himself. Denis Johnson captures this idea nicely with his use of the possessive pronoun to express the exhilaration he felt when it dawned on him and his wife, alone in the wilderness, that "who we were was all we had. . . . We realized our lives before had never before been our own—*our* lives."[7]

Such self-reliance carries with it a tremendous sense of capability, a surge of power and authority, and a sense of responsibility. But the responsibility that is meant here is an individualistic concept, not a social one. It is responsibility for oneself and what one does, not responsibility to others. Social duty, like the rest of society, is absent from the moral world of the Bonanza Hills camp. The responsibility felt there is a lonely one; Denis and Cindy are responsible in the sense that if something goes wrong, they have no one to blame but themselves. It is interesting that in his account Johnson places himself in the company of his wife. Although he is not alone, he might as well be. He makes the couple into a single self by essentially engulfing her identity into his own. He uses the first person plural, but it is the first person singular that we hear. There is a vexing thing about autonomy: it is hard to share.

Autonomy defeats selflessness—not always, but often, and more often today than a generation ago, as pollster Daniel Yankelovich and others have observed. More important than the ordering of values that often ranks autonomy in first place is the way in which other social values come to be understood individualistically and in terms of autonomy. Two illustrations of this interpretive power of autonomy can be seen in the notions of justice and equality.

Justice in the Light of Autonomy

In some extreme societies, such as Singapore, justice means almost exclusively preserving social order. Americans view justice quite differently; for them, it means protecting the rights and respecting the dignity of the individual. "Due process of law" is easy to reconcile with autonomy. Some Americans—quite a few actually—thought it was proper for the Singapore authorities to punish an American teenager for vandalism by caning him. However, many of those who supported the caning there would not support such a policy here. It seems likely that the Singapore authorities were not primarily concerned with conducting a "fair" trial, in our sense of the term: they were concerned not with due process but with deterrence. They used this hapless young man to send a message to their own teenagers and to the international community. Singapore is a community that places obedience and public order at the center of its political philosophy, in the same way that we place autonomy at the center of ours.[8]

"Get-tough" Americans who applauded the caning did not say explicitly which civil liberties they themselves would be ready to give up to have a graffiti-free environment, less threatening public adolescent behavior, and less sheer unruliness: the ban on unreasonable search and seizure? habeas corpus? the right to legal counsel? trial by jury? Autonomy is easy to dismiss when it is somebody else's backside facing the cane.

Equality in the Service of Autonomy

Until recently, equality was fairly easy to reconcile with autonomy because when most Americans spoke of equality, they meant equality of opportunity, not equality of outcome: equal starts, not equal finishes. Autonomy is right at home with the competition, work ethic, and self-reliance that equality of opportunity promotes. On the other hand, after two decades of bureaucratic growth, affirmative action programs are facing a political backlash because they have shifted from equality of opportunity to equality of result. Affirmative action programs are now seen as creating a conflict between equality and autonomy, and Americans are profoundly uncomfortable with that conflict. White males believe that their rights have been violated; some African Americans and Latino/as feel that affirmative action has erased the merit of their individual achievements and eroded the respect they deserve.

Liberal individualism seemed to want it both ways. The original arguments in the civil rights debates focused precisely on the immoral and irrational basis of racial prejudice. Why should skin color differentiate a person any more than hair color, eye color, or stature? Civil rights advocates pleaded for the abandonment of arbitrary stereotyping: "See me as a person, not as an African American, Jew, or woman. Judge me by myself and for myself." This was an autonomy-based argument. Yet affirmative action today does not place the individual self in the forefront but his or her representation as a member of a group. How can the two now be reconciled? Autonomy, the instrument at the center of liberal philosophy, is paradoxically being used to cut the heart out of the liberal agenda.

If affirmative action is to be defended, it is more straightforward, and probably more honest, to do so on the basis of group compensation.[9] One could well argue that African Americans as a group should be given the long end of the stick today because they got the short end yesterday and for three hundred years of North American slavery and discrimination before that. Yet it is hard for Americans to accept giving someone a benefit that he does not necessarily deserve as an individual but nonetheless is entitled to as a member of a group.

Why should it be so difficult? A big part of the reason, we suggest, is that doing so serves neither the autonomy of the beneficiary nor the autonomy of those who lose out. If affirmative action were explicitly justified on the basis of group compensation for past discrimination, then the preferred treatment—the college admission, the job, the promotion, or whatever—would send the message that what is important about those who benefit is their identity as group members, not their unique identity as individuals. Such a message does not respect them as persons; it honors them not as "I's" but only as "they's," and does not promote their autonomy. It may give them resources they can later use to become autonomous; but then again, it may also get them—and others—into a dangerous habit of thinking of themselves as group members first and individuals second, and it may make them dependent upon group benefits. These two habits are nearly as bad as crack cocaine in the eyes of the autonomy-minded.

From the point of view of the losers, on the other hand, affirmative action based on group compensation for past discrimination looks, feels, and tastes like unfair punishment. "I have never personally discriminated against blacks," the white male applicant says, and this may be perfectly true. "So why am I being punished for the sins of my father?" A communally oriented Old Testament morality may be able to accept the governance of a God who visits "iniquity of the fathers upon the children unto the third and fourth generations," but this will not sit well with angry white males.

In a way, though, all affirmative action programs inherently do sacrifice individuals for the sake of society. They represent a contemporary form of retributive justice. They force some individuals to pay a price in order to restore proper order to the moral community, to right an imbalance. They could, and maybe should, be publicly justified in exactly that way.

Such an argument would face a steep uphill climb in the culture of autonomy. Since the eighteenth-century Enlightenment, autonomy has been the bitter enemy of "barbaric" and "premodern" notions of justice like retribution, revenge, and punishment, particularly when applied for the sake of the larger community rather than for the sake of the individual who is being punished. Autonomy is compatible with punishment only for the purposes of deterrence and rehabilitation. Thus Jeremy Bentham, the iconoclastic English legal reformer and the father of utilitarianism, argued in favor of the doctrine of *mens rea* (which requires that the defendant's intention be considered) and against the doctrine of strict liability (which holds that one should be punished for the unlawful consequences of an action regardless of intent). He did so on the grounds that punishing a violator who lacked mental capacity or wrongful intent (as strict liability would do) would have no deterrent effect. The prospect of the electric chair will not deter a murderer who is insane. The prospect of prison time for manslaughter to "deter" a driver who has a sudden heart attack and drives up onto the sidewalk is ludicrous; his action was clearly unintended and therefore requires no deterrence.

Sensible enough. However, Bentham badly underestimated the ubiquitous appeal of revenge and overestimated the power of reason.

Reason does not seem up to the task of suppressing the desire for revenge. Retribution serves the popular sense of rightness and order. We have a deep-seated need to feel ourselves in the presence of order "out there" in the world. This need for order is rooted in the history of our species as well as in the biography of the individual. It begins in knowing that someone is guarding the compound and tending the fire; it begins in the reassuring glow of the nightlight emanating from our parents' bedroom across the hall from the nursery.

Maybe angry white men are correct in feeling that affirmative action programs are unfairly asking them to pay for something that was not their fault. Maybe the moral response should be that restoring balance and moral order to our badly twisted, racist society is more important than fairness to any one individual. One can bring considerable logic to such an argument. But most Americans still will not tolerate premises that negate autonomy, and these conclusions trample it underfoot. Affirmative action that requires more than equality of opportunity is the ultimate enemy of autonomy. Must we choose between autonomy and the values of equal respect, nondiscrimination, equality of result, and what Catholic theologians call the "preferential option for the poor"?

Americans continue to hope that equality of opportunity will be enough to remedy past discrimination and that "color-blind" policies will work—policies that are blind to the primacy of group, race, and class in our lives. By now, however, these policies have proven themselves ineffectual. At the end of the day, Americans want very much *not* to have to choose between autonomy and other big-ticket values like law and order (security), justice, and equality.

Who can blame them? Who among us is ready to step out of the frying pan of individualism and into the fire of a more authoritarian society or, alternatively, a more communitarian one? If it is true that both authoritarian and communitarian impulses are deeply rooted in our psychological natures (as we believe they are), then who among us is ready to abandon the modern Enlightenment dream—Kant's dream certainly, but Freud's dream too—that mankind can tame wild justice and free ourselves, at least to some modest extent, from our natural need for authority and dependence? Autonomy is the waking recollection of that dream. It challenges us to grow up and to be rational. It is humiliating to admit that this challenge may be one we cannot meet.

PUBLIC QUESTIONS, PRIVATE ANSWERS

So highly do Americans value autonomy these days that they either place it above competing values, or insist on defining other values so that they seem not really to conflict with it. A steady diet of such thinking builds a formidable cultural and moral force. Today that force permeates both our public discourse and our private thoughts and feelings.

Consider the public dimension of autonomy. The American understanding of autonomy has affected our public policies and influenced the means we use to change individual behavior and to exercise social control. Several types of cases show the limits of autonomy in public policymaking.

In some cases, conformity to general rules and procedures designed to protect individual autonomy in the abstract leads to particular actions that have perverse consequences, violating our original intentions and our moral common sense. Here "respecting a person's autonomy" in theory is tantamount to disregarding her or his real needs and interests in the here and now of everyday existence. Examples include policies regarding the deinstitutionalization of the mentally ill, the treatment of the homeless, and a person's right to refuse medical care. What these cases have in common is that they all reflect the fact that other people can sometimes see the consequences of our self-destructive personal behavior better than we can ourselves.

In these cases rational persuasion rarely works to overcome self-destructive behavior. Temporary physical restraint is one alternative, although not the only one. (We would argue that it is certainly justifiable at times.) A host of interventions by the caring physician can be brought into play to "bring a patient around." In a social and political atmosphere obsessed with autonomy, however, doctors, social workers, and counselors often stand by and do nothing rather than avert a disaster that they can see coming; they are forced to be more concerned with protecting themselves and their institutions than with their patients. The correct response, we believe, is to reassert moral common sense against autonomy in a way that is pragmatic and geared to particular circumstances.

Even when autonomy does not restrain us from doing the right thing, it may keep us from doing it for the right reasons. This second type of public policy case also demonstrates the limits of autonomy. In the culture of autonomy, public policymakers sometimes coerce individuals to change their behavior (because they believe it is morally right to do so), then justify the coercion by arguing that the old behavior was harmful to others. In fact, that behavior may have been not so much harmful as simply wrong. Policymakers are forced into this deceptive stance by the culture of autonomy, which says, in essence, that public officials are not supposed to make moral judgments in their official capacity; that their sole legitimate job is to protect the public and individuals from harm. In other words, we first purport to find something to be harmful to others, then on that ground label it wrong. In reality, we often first conclude that something is wrong, then seek evidence that it is harmful. Under these circumstances, it is not surprising that "evidence" is sometimes exaggerated or even manufactured.

When it became apparent, for example, that the use of DDT would be an ecological disaster, destroying natural habitats, Americans decided we must stop widespread DDT spraying. But the leaders of underdeveloped countries protested the discontinuation, arguing that DDT could save hundreds of thousands of lives by controlling malaria alone. They were more interested in the survival of their children than in the survival of some endangered species. Then somewhere, somehow, the "knowledge" that DDT is a human carcinogen was widely disseminated. This development shifted the debate and made it a matter of balancing personal and individual benefits, rather than arbitrating between conflicting claims of the individual and the environment.[10] In fact, there was (and still is) no clear evidence that DDT is a specific carcinogen for human beings.

It is important to understand how the concept of autonomy paints public policy discourse into this awkward and dishonest corner. Such policy dilemmas are frequently found in the field of public health, especially health risks that are related to personal behavior and lifestyle. In order to protect the autonomy of HIV-positive individuals, AIDS was purposely not listed as a venereal disease, even though it is clearly, though not exclusively, so. There are laws on the books for mandatory testing for syphilis and gonorrhea. But American policymakers preferred protecting the privacy of the individual to preventing the spread of the disease.

Oftentimes autonomy makes us overlook the valid interests of society when they conflict with the interests and choices of individuals. This is a third domain of public policy where the moral value of autonomy must be carefully assessed. This situation frequently arises in making decisions about the use of life-sustaining medical treatment and the care of the dying. Can medical treatment desired by patients and their families ever be denied in a morally defensible way in order to serve justice and the needs of others? What if the treatment asked for is inordinately expensive? If autonomy means giving a patient a right to refuse medical treatment, does it also mean giving the patient the right to demand treatment?

Or taking the logic of autonomy one step further, does it mean the patient has a right to active assistance with committing suicide? Should physician-assisted suicide and euthanasia be legalized, or can autonomy be overridden here in the name of competing social values and interests? These social values include respecting the sanctity of life, protecting those who are vulnerable to medical abuse and neglect, and maintaining the ethical and professional integrity of the medical profession, which since ancient times has pledged never intentionally to kill. This topic is discussed more fully in chapters 11 and 12.

Autonomy effects the way we ask questions and define issues in the political arena, but it also lives and works closer to home. To appreciate its affect on private morality, we suggest that the reader reflect on these questions:

- What does it mean to be a member of society today and of the various subgroups that compose it? Does "membership" suggest to you any deep affiliations or commitments in any of the spheres of your life? How important is it to you to be a member of a political entity, such as a country? A civic group? A religious tradition? An economic enterprise, like a firm or a company? A family? Is it possible to have a deep sense of membership in one or two of these spheres but not in the others?

- How do you experience social ties, obligations, and the expectations of others? As stifling constraints? As necessary inconveniences, accepted begrudgingly because you realize that your own self-interest is served when everyone accepts these limitations? As valid moral duties imposed upon you from outside, but not as truly emanating from your own will or as authentically expressive of who you are as a unique person?

- What does it mean to be a unique individual, a self, a free agent, a person? And how should society stand in relation to that self? Do the values of society set the purposes of the self, or vice versa?

Are social relationships basically means to personal ends? Is self-identity inherited, discovered, or created?

Who am I? Where do I stand? What really matters? The answers people give to these questions determine how they experience freedom in their everyday lives. These questions are not simply conceptual issues of moral theory; they have to do with the character and quality of practical everyday life. They have to do with the patterns of moral thinking and feeling that American culture—the culture of autonomy—makes readily available today.

In his comprehensive study of survey research on American values conducted in the 1970s and early 1980s, Daniel Yankelovich documented what he called a transition from an "ethic of self-denial" to an "ethic of self-fulfillment." He paraphrases the ethic of self-denial in the following terms: "I give hard work, loyalty and steadfastness. I swallow my frustrations and suppress my impulse to do what I would enjoy, and do what is expected of me instead. I do not put myself first; I put the needs of others ahead of my own. I give a lot, but what I get in return is worth it."[11]

Attitudes and values like these, he believes, have been the basis of the goals of American society since World War II. But they are presently shifting like geological plates in a slow but irreversible cultural change toward a refusal to sacrifice personal growth and fulfillment in the name of conventional expectations, institutions, and responsibilities. Yankelovich continues: "The ethics of the search for self-fulfillment discard many of the traditional rules of personal conduct. They permit more sexual freedom, for example, and they put less emphasis on sacrifice 'for its own sake.' In their extreme form, the new rules simply turn the old ones on their head, and in place of the old self-denial ethic we find people who refuse to deny *anything* to themselves—not out of bottomless appetite, but on the strange moral principle that 'I have a duty to myself.' "[12]

What Yankelovich describes here is not precisely autonomy, perhaps, but autonomy and self-fulfillment as a philosophy of life have a close affinity with each other. The social attitudes that reject self-denial create a climate that fosters the proliferation of autonomy and rights claims. With those claims comes an estrangement of the self from the rules, structures, and relationships that actually defined the self in an earlier era. Social responsibilities impinge upon and "repress" the self in the new ethics of autonomy and self-fulfillment. And in their private lives people are less and less willing to pay the price of self-denial—whether it be to avoid divorce, keep within one's budget, practice responsible family planning, give up anonymous and promiscuous sex, put the kids through college, give up your job to follow your husband, split the difference and look for a compromise, or slip and fall on your neighbor's sidewalk and say it was your fault. As for people who are still willing to pay the price of self-denial (and of course many still are, or else we wouldn't have a functioning society at all), they may look at others around them who are not and feel like suckers. Resentment born of ambivalence about self-sacrifice and self-denial in a culture that no longer publicly esteems these virtues is building to dangerous levels.

Writing in 1981, Yankelovich was rather sanguine about this transition. He noticed that the ethic of self-fulfillment was placing considerable strain on the social fabric and social institutions, but it was only a transitional phase, he argued, and American society was on its way toward a third philosophy of life, which he called "the ethic of commitment." This ethic would combine what is most valid in the individualism of rights and autonomy, with an acknowledgment of social interests and responsibilities. Today, we see little evidence of this synthesis. On the contrary, in the intervening years the pendulum has continued to swing in the direction of the "moral freedom" that sociologist Alan Wolfe has found in his interview studies and research.

THE BACK OF THE BUS

The public and private dimensions of the culture of autonomy are nicely illustrated by the following incident. Rockland County, a suburban area about thirty miles north of New York City, is the home of a large community of ultra-orthodox Hasidic Jews. Every morning Hasidic men board a commuter bus bound for the city, and they conduct their morning prayers en route. Their religious traditions and practices dictate a strict separation between men and women during prayers, and they have affixed a sliding curtain around several seats so they can close themselves off from other passengers. This custom has been going on for some time, with the cooperation of the bus company and the drivers.

One morning in 1993 a controversy that would be hard to imagine outside the American culture of autonomy broke out. A woman passenger on the bus was asked to change her seat so that more men could position themselves behind the curtain. She refused. Tempers flared, words were exchanged. The bus pulled over near the Lincoln Tunnel (appropriately enough) and the Hasidim stepped off the bus to complete their prayers. Sima Rabinovicz, the irate woman, herself a Soviet Jewish immigrant and a feminist, claimed she had been threatened and intimidated, and she subsequently switched to another bus line. She brought a formal complaint with the New York State Division of Human Rights and threatened a civil suit in which she was to be represented by the New York Civil Liberties Union. Newspaper coverage revealed simmering tensions between the Orthodox community in Rockland and their less observant and more secular neighbors. More than a year later, an out-of-court settlement was reached in which the bus company would no longer put up a curtain to separate men at prayer from female passengers; but if no riders on the bus objected, and if it did not violate safety codes, Hasidic men would be able to put up their own cloth barrier and carry on with their worship.

A social accommodation, mutually arrived at and quietly practiced, is always vulnerable to the complaint that it violates an individual's rights, and it is very fragile when exposed to the harsh klieg lights of legal debate. The bus company is owned and operated by a Hasidic family business, but it is publicly licensed and receives state subsidies. Questions were raised about whether a public conveyance should be permitted to display religious symbols or to allow religious services on board. The practice of religion— a public, communal work in the eyes of most faiths, but a private act among consenting adults in the eyes of the Constitution and public policy— could not infringe upon the public domain, no more on public buses than in public schools. Moreover, the exclusion of women is discriminatory, particularly in so graphic and symbolic a way, involving curtains and bus seats. "I didn't move because I didn't feel it was right just because I'm a woman for them to tell me what to do," Rabinovicz was quoted as saying afterward. "Today, they can tell me to move my seat; tomorrow, they will tell me to get off the bus. And they can tell me those things just because I'm a woman. Nothing else."[13]

Not lost on any of the participants in this dispute was the legacy of Rosa Parks and her refusal to give up her seat and move to the back of the bus in Montgomery, Alabama, at a very different time and in a very different place but for apparently identical reasons. Finding this symbolic resonance too attractive to resist, an attorney defending the bus company and the Hasidic group also cast the dispute in civil libertarian terms. "We think it's a perfect metaphor for religious liberty," said Kevin J. Hasson of the Becket Fund for Religious Liberty. "The religious people not only got sent to the back of the bus, but got kicked off the bus."[14]

How do such things get so blown out of proportion? A simple act of everyday courtesy—"Would you mind changing your seat? Thank you"— becomes a matter of sexism and religious freedom. It ends in year-long litigation, the state's human rights bureaucracy steps in, and advocacy groups clash. Right versus right. We take our quarrel to the Constitution— the Nanny State—when we can't get along.

It might be said that this incident reveals what a litigious society we have become, and so we have; or that it reveals our tendency to flaunt our ethnic differences rather than mute them, and so it does. We have become an In Your Face society. However, explanations like these leave something out as well. James Q. Wilson, in *The Moral Sense*, remarks that "The idea of autonomous individuals choosing everything—their beliefs and values, their history and traditions, their social forms and family structures—is a vainglorious idea, one that could be invented only by thinkers who felt compelled to construct society out of theories."[15]

Wilson is certainly correct that it is foolish to use autonomy to explain how societies historically originated and actually function. But he leaves unanswered the philosophical question of autonomy's adequacy as a moral ideal of how people *ought* to live. We share his impatience with abstract theories, especially those that attempt to reduce everything to a single value or principle, be it happiness, efficiency, or freedom. But his observation is misleading in two ways.

First, the idea of autonomy does not come only—or even mainly— from the writings of social theorists; it derives from the recognition of the biological uniqueness of our species; it grows out of the lived experience of struggles for rights and recognition that have engaged countless millions of people for three hundred years. Closer to home, the autonomy being asserted on the Rockland bus was a direct offshoot of the civil rights struggles of the past three decades. Political theories (the important ones that we can still learn from, at any rate) do not spin concepts out of whole cloth; they articulate aspirations that are implicit in institutions and in social behavior. Theory is a way of articulating those things implicit in the activities and relationships of social life.

The second way Wilson's observation is misleading involves the extent to which our thoughts and feelings in America today have become theory driven. "Vainglorious" it may be, but autonomy now preoccupies the American scene. It permeates our social discourse; in moral discourse we can talk of little else besides rights, freedom, respect, and empowerment. Even more, it permeates our social and personal style, where everything has become a matter of "principle." Honest differences are not recognized; the character and morality of one's opponent must be impugned. Compromise, accommodation, and public affirmations of ambiguity, even indecision, are taken as signs of weakness.

People with sharp elbows need a lot of elbow room. The trouble is, the bus we are all on in America today is getting very crowded, and people are not prone to give up either their seats or their "space." Perhaps it is time we started thinking as much about what holds us together as about what sets us apart; as much about our manner of living together (our "manners," morals, and character) as about our autonomy and rights.

4

Seduced by Autonomy: Heeding the Grand Inquisitor and Other Critics

And if I am for myself alone, what then am I?
—HILLEL, Babylonian Talmud, *Aboth* I:14

CREATING A SOCIETY in which autonomy flourishes has been one of America's greatest achievements. At the same time, the preeminence given to autonomy today poses one of our gravest dangers. This paradox can be resolved by grasping a simple but elusive truth: there can be no free society without individual autonomy, yet no sustainable society can rest on autonomy alone.

The component ideas of autonomy—individual rights, freedom of choice, privacy, independence, freedom from outside interference—are viewed as having great moral legitimacy. They express deeply felt aspirations and worthy ideals. At the same time, other principles that remind us of our social natures and our interdependence as human beings—community, citizenship, authority, obligation, responsibility, reciprocity, tradition, rules, limits—also have great resonance. They are the words of civilization and moral order; they are the elements of an essential vision of the human good. In fact, we perceive them as indispensable, because they are firmly rooted in our psychological natures. These ideas derive from the fact that the human identity is shaped by—and the human good is lived within and through—social roles (such as being a parent), relationships (such as providing care), and institutional structures (such as the family and civic and religious groups).

No political or moral discourse is adequate to the richness of human moral experience if it lacks either vocabulary: the vocabulary of autonomy or community. It is critical that we retain what is of enduring value in the language of rights and autonomy, but it is no less critical that we sustain the language of responsibilities and relationships. If there is a danger inherent in the political imagination of Americans today—and we are convinced that the danger is serious—it comes from an excessive emphasis on autonomy and too little appreciation of human interdependence and mutual responsibility. To redress that imbalance and to restore a better equilibrium between autonomy and social control, we must draw on the wisdom contained in more relational understandings of human nature, human flourishing, and the social good.

Our humanity is fulfilled by conjoining rights and responsibilities, autonomy and relationships, independence and interdependence. The tools of each are essential to being and becoming the kind of creatures we are. How each of us as an individual and how our society as a whole understands the connection between these two poles of our moral being is therefore of crucial significance. Getting this connection right is crucial to how successful a society will be in solving its problems and getting things done. It is also crucial to the morale of a society, to how its people feel about the way they have accomplished their goals.

We live now with this paradox. Despite autonomy's central place in the American moral imagination, most of the critics of autonomy today seem to come from the conservative end of the cultural spectrum. On the left, where one might expect to find more communitarian and collectivist points of view, the language of libertarianism and liberation has virtually taken over. The intellectual "new" left, based now almost entirely in university and academic settings and having no significant political constituency of its own, has displaced the "old" left of the labor movement and working-class solidarity. It is characteristic of the new left to focus on lifestyle and identity issues more than on gritty, frustrating issues such as unemployment, job training, and the redistribution of wealth and power.

Since the 1960s, the new left has embraced autonomy every bit as tightly as right-wing libertarianism. In the "identity issues" that now consume its energies—racial and gender discrimination, multiculturalism, sexual orientation, abortion, freedom of expression, and the like—the new left has found common cause with mainstream liberals who disagree with leftists on questions of economic policy. What holds these strange ideological bedfellows together in this bewildering transitional period is the ideal of autonomy.

On the right, however, matters are even more volatile and complex. Cultural libertarians and free-market economic conservatives form one camp, whereas cultural conservatives, religious fundamentalists, and blue-collar populists, who have shifted from the Democratic to the Republican party in vast numbers since the Reagan landslide of 1980, form an opposing coalition.

The balance between individual autonomy and social control, between personal rights and moral responsibilities, is the primary cause of this major schism in American politics. Important figures on the culturally conservative side of the debate have been scholars such as Gertrude Himmelfarb, James Q. Wilson, Hilton Kramer, and the late Allan Bloom, as well as public figures such as William Bennett, the former secretary of education in the Reagan administration. Numerous influential religious leaders keep hammering away at the excesses of rights and autonomy, even as conservative think tanks and numerous conservative public interest law firms unfurl the banner of autonomy as they march toward deregulated industry and curtailed paternalistic federal welfare policies. Many Republican political leaders personify the dilemma of trying to support the culture of autonomy, with its entrepreneurial individualism, and a religious and cultural revitalization movement that is profoundly dissatisfied with autonomy.

It may be easier to understand the situation by taking a look at the causes of the conflict. Historically, the conflict between autonomy and social order was seen as a struggle between the needs and passions of the individual and the order necessary to ensure the stability of the state or the authority of the church. Freedom and autonomy hung in the balance of this debate. Liberty was often interpreted as a direct threat to social order. Two of the great and passionate defenses of order were articulated by William Shakespeare and Fyodor Dostoyevsky. (Discussed below.)

This polarity, however, is no longer appropriate. Instead, it can be reconciled by broadening it to include other elements in addition to the defenseless individual and the powerful state. We must distinguish among the different spheres of society within which autonomy can operate, and this will inevitably shift the moral argument.

The question of social spheres is significant because autonomy is more appropriate in some parts of society and in some parts of our personal lives than in others. It properly guides moral life in some spheres but misdirects it in others. Our argument is that autonomy works best in the sphere of politics, where it protects the individual against the misuse of government power. However, when it is extended into the domains of civic and family life, treating all relationships as power relationships, autonomy often leads to morally blind and inappropriate conclusions. (This point will be developed in later chapters, particularly in chapter 9, where we distinguish among the social spheres of the political state, the market, civil society, and the family.) Bounded autonomy is a precious human and historical achievement; blanket autonomy is an unsustainable pipe dream. Blanket coercion is a totalitarian nightmare, historically all-too-common; bounded coercion is the linchpin of social order and one of the conditions that make it possible for society to be a place of individual freedom and human flourishing.

THE DEFENDERS OF ORDER

The defenders of order usually direct their criticism of the culture of autonomy along one of two lines. One such line, developed by the theologian Stanley Hauerwas, is that autonomy is morally flabby because it is little more than an ethic of selfishness and self-indulgence. In a similar expression of the same kind of criticism, sociologist Daniel Bell decried what he called the dominant "hedonism" behind the cultural transformations begun in the late 1960s.[1]

The second line of criticism of the culture of autonomy is that the widespread deference accorded to autonomy today in the law and in secular morality threatens to undermine the moral order itself. A spate of books published in the 1990s developed this theme. Robert Hughes, in *Culture of Complaint* ridicules an atmosphere in which excessive autonomy breeds a pervasive sense of victimhood and personal complaint. This temperament, in turn, distracts us from common problems of much greater importance and hamstrings our capacity to develop a communal or democratic response to these problems. Symbolism triumphs over substance, gridlock prevails, and opportunities for mutual accommodation are missed.[2]

In an analysis along similar lines, political theorist Jean Bethke Elshtain argues in *Democracy on Trial* that the sense of civic culture vital to a working democracy is undermined by libertarians of the right and multiculturalists and radical feminists of the left. These groups practice what Elshtain calls a "politics of displacement," which destroys a proper ordering in society made up of boundaries between the public and private spheres. Thus sexual orientation is turned into a political identity demanding equal rights and respect, and elections to high office center not on the candidate's public policy positions but on the presence or absence of private scandal.[3]

These works focus on the effects of the culture of autonomy on our sense of community and our frayed social fabric. Other critiques zero in on the functioning of important social institutions, feeling that our passion for equality is undermining the very institutions essential to the flourishing—indeed the survival—of the individual. William A. Henry III, author of *In Defense of Elitism*, squarely pits equality against excellence and says that for the past thirty years equality has been consistently winning. Henry provides a provocative indictment of the social costs and stupidity of America's recent preoccupation with equality, as though it could possibly be achieved in isolation from other equally precious attributes of democracy. This preoccupation, he argues, has not achieved much real equality for disadvantaged people, nor any significant redistribution of wealth from top to bottom. The egalitarian philosophy has stripped our leading institutions of the work ethic and high standards they require to function effectively in an increasingly competitive post–cold war world.[4]

A similar indictment is found in Philip K. Howard's *The Death of Common Sense: How Law Is Suffocating America*. Howard directs his ire at economic inefficiency caused by excessive governmental regulation and the general litigiousness of a society preoccupied with individual rights and demands.[5]

We have singled out these books because the authors have all put their respective fingers on something worrisome about our culture: they question who we, as a people, have become in the United States. They expose a surly individualism, a disposition on the part of aggrieved individuals to make excessive and unreasonable demands on social institutions.

Moreover, all these works have in common a sense of moral disorder, not normlessness or anomie. Claims to rights and demands for dignity and respect, no matter how well deserved, are overloading the system. They are killing something—call it toleration, cooperation, consensus, pragmatism, striving for achievement, teamwork, or common sense—essential to social order in this country and that has contributed mightily to the success of the American experiment.

This sense of disorder and the need to respond aggressively to it is captured in the very titles or subtitles of many of these works: the "fraying of America" (Hughes's subtitle), "on trial" "defense" "death," and "suffocating America." In other works, America is being "de-moralized" (Gertrude Himmelfarb) or "disunited" (Arthur Schlesinger, Jr.).[6]

Let us consider the relationship between autonomy and social order more carefully. The charge that autonomy is little more than selfishness is mistaken. Autonomy is not an ethic of selfishness, nor is self-indulgence the same as rational self-fulfillment. As we earlier defined it, autonomy means freedom from outside restraint and the freedom to live one's own life in one's own way. To be autonomous is to live by your own law, or only by laws that you have embraced and accepted as your own. It is to be self-sovereign. It is to be the author of your life, your self, and your actions. Nothing in these notions necessitates selfishness or egoism. Self-determining conduct need not be exclusively self-serving. Being the author of your own life says nothing per se about the moral content of that life.

As an ethic, autonomy means living according to your own values and principles, as these are refined in the light of informed, rational deliberation and settled conviction. This ethic is a far cry from an anything-goes, do-your-own-thing morality. There is no obvious reason that an autonomous person cannot identify with principles of justice and moral virtue. Not only is autonomy compatible with just and altruistic ideals, it seems to go naturally with them. The free and secure person is a more open and charitable person. It is insecurity about one's worth that often breeds defensiveness and hostility.

Although autonomy is not an ideal of selfishness or disorderly self-indulgence, it is always self-centered, self-expressive, and individualistic. It can be—according to most philosophers it *must* be—based on rational will rather than license, and it is the self's reason, not that of a community or a higher authority. Autonomy's mood is always possessive. It speaks in the first person singular rather than the first person plural. It is a vision of free *I*'s, not free *We*'s.

What about the charge that autonomy undermines social order? This is not simply an empirical claim that some of the problems and disorders that exist in society today are products of our love affair with autonomy. The indictment runs deeper than that. It is a philosophical claim that there is some basic incompatibility between the very idea of autonomy and human nature, or the requirements of social order, or both.

In one sense that claim is mistaken, yet it contains an important insight. The defenders of order are wrong to focus solely on autonomy's rejection of external authority. In doing so they overlook the fact that it is primarily through the internalization of such authority during childhood that social order is sustained and transmitted from one generation to the next. A much more fundamental criticism can be made of autonomy when it becomes the dominant value orientation in a society. Autonomy is no more antithetical to social order than is authoritarianism or communitarianism. Autonomy in fact relies on the type of social order that comes from processes of socialization and the internalization of social norms and restraints, particularly during childhood and adolescence.

The problem with the culture of autonomy is that an overemphasis on autonomy in a culture undermines those very mechanisms of socialization, and the development of the social emotions of guilt, shame, pride, and conscience, upon which a society that allows wide latitude for personal freedom relies. These social emotions and the bases of self-restraint may break down if the social institutions of family and civil society that support them break down. If that happens, social order can be maintained by resorting to more primitive emotions, such as fear, but that means relying on political mechanisms that are more authoritarian than anyone wants. Our analysis, therefore, turns the traditional reactionary and antiliberal critique of autonomy on its head. Instead of leading to social chaos and breakdown, excessive autonomy and individualism are more likely to lead eventually to increased repression and authoritarianism.

Internalizing social norms is the key to liberal social order. We become capable, functional members of a human moral community as a result of the childrearing and educational practices that socialize us. Socialization occurs when individuals internalize the norms and expectations of the broader society—mediated through their parents and other adults—and make them their own. Every human society relies on socialization, on the knowledge that people can and must internalize the rules that make cooperation and stability possible. Once individuals have made those rules their own, most people obey most of the rules, cooperate, and conform most of the time voluntarily. They do so out of habit, without consciously thinking about what they are doing, because it seems natural and right.

When peasants from the French Protestant village of Le Chambon, who sheltered Jewish refugees during the Nazi occupation, were asked why they would risk their own safety to help others, they could scarcely understand the question. How could they not help?, they wondered. What other way is there to live?[7] We feel comfortable obeying the external rules that we have internalized because by internalizing them they have become a part of "us." Following these internalized norms feels like, and in fact is, an affirmation of our self-identity.

No society can sustain itself for very long if it has to maintain social order by having a policeman on every corner all the time. Surveillance and external coercion are inefficient and expensive. External coercion is only a supplemental tool of social order. Societies survive by putting a policeman—and an ego ideal—inside almost every head.

Socialization and internalization are the linchpins that hold bounded autonomy and liberal social order together in a delicate balance. Behind the socialization process itself stands the very way we are put together as human beings, our biological prematurity, frailty, and dependence; our psychological makeup; our linguistic and symbol-utilizing capacities; our culture-making and culture-bearing natures.

Traditional critics of autonomy have a second point to score, and here they are on more solid ground. They sense how impossibly heavy a burden the ideal of autonomy places on human rationality, and how strained is the human capacity to face the terrifying fact of our own freedom. These more substantive criticisms were articulated by two of our most psychologically astute commentators on the human condition and its paradoxes, Shakespeare and Dostoyevsky.

The English playwright and the Russian novelist shared the powerful insight that the ideal of autonomy is at odds with powerful and fundamental opposing psychological forces. For Shakespeare, what we today call autonomy would inevitably unleash a psychological chain reaction that would destroy our very humanity. For Dostoyevsky, autonomy, which he explicitly identified with the radical philosophy of spiritual freedom offered by Jesus, is fundamentally incompatible with man's rebellious but childlike and authority-craving nature. These two authors profoundly influenced Sigmund Freud, who laid the groundwork for our modern understanding of human nature and human conduct.

THE COUNSEL OF ULYSSES

Europeans living in the early seventeenth century were caught between two worlds. One of these, the hierarchical, status-conscious world of medieval feudalism and monarchy, was the world of the past. The other, the individualistic modern world of Enlightenment, commerce, and democracy, was the world of the future. It was a confusing time in which to live, and it was a particularly uncomfortable and perplexing time to be an intellectual. The modern worldview had developed sufficiently that those with sensitive eyes could see its radical implications, but it was far from clear what kind of new society would emerge once the old order had been swept away.

The poet John Donne was one of the unsettled ones. He captured the conservative sensibility of the time precisely:

And new Philosophy calls all in doubt . . .
'Tis all in peeces, all cohaerence gone;
All just supply, and all Relation:
Prince, Subject, Father, Sonne, are things forgot,
For every man alone thinkes he hath got
To be a Phoenix, and that then can bee
None of that kinde, of which he is, but hee.[8]

Donne's nightmare has become our waking reality. Most of the ingredients for the culture of autonomy are contained in these lines—individualism, the quest for self-expression, a sense of uniqueness apart from one's position in a larger social structure—in a word, autonomy rampant. Donne saw the demise of a moral order that had maintained "coherence" and "relation" by keeping individuals in their (hierarchically ordered) places, whether in political or familial roles. For every person to be a phoenix (a mythological bird that is consumed by fire, only to be reborn from its own ashes) would be to deny our common humanity. It is a dangerous and impossible conceit.

What Donne described, Shakespeare analyzed. One of Shakespeare's most philosophical statements on the problem of order comes in the marvelous speech on degree by Ulysses in Troilus and Cressida. In this scene the Greek heroes are in council before the walls of Troy, pondering what to do about Achilles's assertion of individuality in abandoning the common cause—his assertion of autonomy, we might say. He was refusing to help the Greek war effort any longer because the leader of the Greek expedition, Agamemnon, had offended him by taking a slave girl that Achilles considered rightfully his. Should the Greek heroes succumb to the primacy of individual desires over the needs of the group, Ulysses warns, a fundamental disorder will be set loose in the world:

> . . . Oh, when degree is shak'd,
> Which is the ladder to all high designs,
> The enterprise is sick! How could communities,
> Degrees in schools and brotherhoods in cities,
> Peaceful commerce from dividable shores,
> The primogenitive and due of birth,
> Prerogative of age, crowns sceptres laurels,
> But by degree stand in authentic place?
> Take but degree away, untune that string,
> And, hark, what discord follows! each thing meets
> In mere oppugnancy: the bounded waters
> Should lift their bosoms higher than the shores
> And make a sop of all this solid globe:
> Strength should be lord to imbecility,
> And the rude son should strike his father dead:
> Force should be right; or, rather, right and wrong,—
> Between whose endless jar justice resides,—
> Should lose their names, and so should justice too.
> Then everything includes itself in power,
> Power into will, will into appetite;
> And appetite, an universal wolf,
> So doubly seconded with will and power,
> Must make perforce an universal prey,
> And last eat up himself.[9]

It is characteristic of Shakespeare to import contemporary ideas into his treatment of classical material, as this passage surely does. It captures a worldview that was quite conventional and commonplace in the late medieval and early modern period.

Like Donne and other writers of the period, Shakespeare here places social and political relationships squarely in the context of the "Great Chain of Being," an order that permeates all levels of being, from the stars to the affairs of men.[10] This cosmic ordering makes being itself possible, and it alone stands in the way of chaos. Order is fragile, and its maintenance a constant task, for just as heavenly events can affect human affairs on earth, so too can disorder in human doings shake nature itself in its very being.

Thus, in the early seventeenth-century worldview social order is continuous with the natural world, mirroring and participating in it. The hierarchical order of things has priority over the things themselves. Relationships, patterns, and connections are more important than the individual beings connected. Healthy form, the larger social and natural "enterprise," takes precedence over the actions or the agents operating within it.

This is a stern and somewhat threatening picture of the world. To modern eyes, it is jarring to see relationships and structures so uncompromisingly privileged over the persons who are living in them. This aristocratic and traditionalist social order (with its reinforcing theology and cosmology) would be precisely what the modern cultural and political revolutions—the Renaissance and the Reformation, capitalism, scientific materialism, constitutionalism, and liberalism—would overthrow. Liberation in the modern sense meant precisely shaking those degrees, cracking and rending the married calm of states from their fixture. It is a world well lost.

Although we accept the overthrow of the cosmology implicit in Shakespeare's vision, we should not be so quick to dismiss his moral psychology and its warning. Human nature, no less than other aspects of nature, needs some order, pattern, and stability if it is to flourish or even survive. If it is unacceptable to the modern moral imagination to reassert the primacy of relationships over persons; if we can no longer morally stomach the primacy of preexisting customs, roles, and obligations over the will and desired projects of individuals, then we nonetheless need to think hard—much harder than we have in recent years—about the wisdom of merely reversing these propositions and turning Shakespeare's vision on its head.

We need this rethinking for precisely the reason Shakespeare gave. In the absence of relationships, agents have no external or social bearing or purpose; the motivation for their actions must come solely from within.

Without roles, human actions have no point beyond sheer self-expression. Without structures like communities and without harmony, social being is reduced to meetings or encounters of sheer "oppugnancy." These problems emerge when individuals cast off (or are stripped by circumstances of) the social institutions, the symbolic patterns of meaning, and the psychological controls that normally structure their conduct; when they are solely dependent on and accountable to their inner strengths and resources; when they are thrown back, that is to say, into autonomy.

If we take seriously what Shakespeare and other moralists and philosophers have said, we must question the modern assumption that autonomy leads automatically to freedom and human self-realization. What frightened Shakespeare most was not the specific disordering of conventional social relationships: that the young would lord it over the old; that children would disrespect (or even attack) their parents; or that mediocrity and stupidity would roll over excellence and distinction like the flood waters over the land. These particular kinds of disorder are certainly routine and commonplace enough in contemporary society, and we suspect they were not unknown in Elizabethan England either. No, the deeper problem on Shakespeare's mind seems to have been the breakdown of those *fundamental* structures—such as meaningful moral discourse itself—that are preconditions of social order as such. This breakdown is what we are now seeing in modern life.

Many people believe that the ultimate moral degradation of society occurs when might becomes right, when the law of the stronger supplants the law of justice. This was not Shakespeare's point. He acknowledged this danger, but then called attention to a more profound danger. Might may be considered right at a given time, but as long as the idea of right remains viable, the possibility remains open that the idea of right will be attached in some future to behaviors and qualities other than force and physical strength. But what if the very idea of right is lost? What if the structure of a common, traditional moral language is unavailable to each individual in society? Then right, wrong, and justice would "lose their names."

If human beings were unable to use moral names or categories, they would be incapable of shaping and conforming their behavior to *any* outside standards or models. In such a morally mute world, power would be neither right nor wrong, but simply power per se. The modern self's journey to the interior—the inward turn of the modern social imagination so important to the culture of autonomy—would become not a voyage of self-discovery and self-reclamation, like Baby Suggs crossing the Ohio River to freedom, but a nightmare descent from power, to will, to the self-consuming appetite that Shakespeare so stunningly evokes (echoing Saint Paul's warning in Galatians) in the concluding lines of Ulysses' speech: "And appetite, an universal wolf,/ So doubly seconded with will and power,/ Must make perforce an universal prey/And last eat up himself."

ANSWERING THE GRAND INQUISITOR

Writing in the 1860s and 1870s, Fyodor Dostoyevsky had an advantage over Shakespeare: He could see, in Europe and North America, the fruits of the modern world. Autonomy was no longer a fledgling idea in his day but a dominant cultural force. Yet, like Shakespeare, Dostoyevsky was writing in a transitional situation, for being Russian, he was living in a largely medieval and feudal society. In czarist Russia the principles of liberalism, autonomy, and Enlightenment, long since accepted in England, France, and the United States, were still considered radical and subversive. Indeed, modernity would not catch up to Russia until 1917, and it would not last long even then, for by the 1930s Stalin would reimpose an authoritarian state, not unlike the one that had imprisoned Dostoyevsky a century earlier.

In his great novel *The Brothers Karamazov*, Dostoyevsky captured the spiritual and intellectual dilemmas of his age within the microcosm of one extraordinary family. The famous chapter titled "The Grand Inquisitor" is a story told by Ivan Karamazov to his younger brother Alexei. Ivan is a disillusioned rationalist who has lost his faith in both God and the Enlightenment. Alexei, a devout novice monk, is a young man of quite different temperament. "The Grand Inquisitor" involves the sudden return of Christ, who appears in Seville during the height of the Inquisition. No sooner does he arrive than he brings a dead child back to life and attracts an immediate following. The Grand Inquisitor, a ninety-year-old man who is all-powerful in the city, observes this, knows instinctively that this man is Christ, and promptly has him arrested.

Late that night the Inquisitor visits Christ in his dungeon cell and engages in an extended monologue (Christ does not speak) in which he condemns Christ's gospel of freedom and defends the authoritarian rule of the church. The Inquisitor initially intends to execute Christ, but he eventually turns him out into the night instead, admonishing him to return to heaven and leave well enough alone on earth. The sequence is laced with irony and ambiguity so that it is impossible to say whose views the Inquisitor represents: Ivan's or Dostoyevsky's. For our purposes here, it does not matter. We will treat the Inquisitor's speech, as it has often been treated, as a philosophical argument that is significant in its own right.

The Inquisitor interprets Christ's teaching in much the way Saint Paul did. Christ offered mankind a new kind of freedom and asked only that individuals open themselves to that freedom and rise to the responsibility of accepting it. This is the Inquisitor's brilliant interpretation of the significance of Jesus' refusal of Satan's three temptations in the wilderness—his refusal to turn stones into bread, his refusal to cast himself down from the precipice and tempt God, and his refusal to accept the worldly dominion and political authority that Satan offered him.

By refusing to make bread, Jesus was rejecting an appeal to the material needs of the people. He would not bribe his followers; their faith must be autonomously given, not bought. By refusing to save his own life, Jesus was rejecting the authority of the miraculous. Moreover, by rejecting political power, Jesus was refusing to give men a common authority to bow down to.

The Inquisitor argues that Christian freedom asks too much of human nature, which is rebellious and much too weak to bear the burden of true freedom. He justifies the introduction of the authority of the Roman Catholic Church as a replacement for Jewish law and Christian freedom:

> There is no more ceaseless or tormenting care for man, as long as he remains free, than to find someone to bow down to as soon as possible. . . . You knew . . . this essential mystery of human nature, but you rejected the only absolute banner . . . the banner of earthly bread; and you rejected it in the name of freedom and heavenly bread. . . . You desired the free love of man, that he should follow you freely, seduced and captivated by you. Instead of the firm ancient law, man had henceforth to decide for himself, with a free heart, what is good and what is evil, having only your image before him as a guide—but did it not occur to you that he would eventually

reject and dispute even your image and your truth if he was oppressed by so terrible a burden as freedom of choice?[11]

The historical church, in contrast to Christ's original and authentic gospel, has understood this human need, the Inquisitor continues. It has created a comforting and orderly authority, with the illusion of freedom. In this respect the church is acting more compassionately, more lovingly, the Inquisitor insists, than Christ. Finally, the Inquisitor maintains that Christ's experiment with freedom, like modernity's experiment with autonomy and rational Enlightenment, will fail, and human nature will return society to the higher priorities, or more basic needs, of security, material desire, stability, and order: "Oh, we [the church] will convince them that they will only become free when they resign their freedom to us, and submit to us. Will we be right, do you think, or will we be lying? They themselves will be convinced that we are right, for they will remember to what horrors of slavery and confusion your freedom led them."[12]

Shakespeare's Ulysses has reminded us of the dangers inherent in the misuse of autonomy. Autonomy gives individuals a moral liberation from the authority of preexisting rules, roles, and relationships, from inherited and imposed obligations, and from social controls and influences on motivation and behavior. Will individuals so liberated then neglect the moral relationships that remain essential to the human good, leading to the descent from autonomy (self-control) to willfulness (self-indulgence) to self-consuming appetite that Shakespeare feared? Or will they embrace those relationships in a new way, both exercising and controlling their autonomy pragmatically, thus recognizing the moral limits of autonomy— and the moral justification of coercion—when necessary? To heed the counsel of Ulysses, we need to find a path to the second of these possibilities so that we can avoid the first.

The Grand Inquisitor's challenge is somewhat different. Even without the slippery slope from liberty to license, self-control is too hard and too terrible for human nature to bear. The modern ethic of autonomy is itself perverse and immoral, not just because it can be abused, and not just because it leads to violence and disorder, but because it is fundamentally unnatural; it is ontologically inappropriate, out of keeping with our human being, and therefore cruel and immoral.

We need not subscribe to the Inquisitor's dark view of freedom or to his pessimistic appraisal of human nature to accept the power of his position. To avoid his discouraging conclusions, however, we must look more closely at human nature. For within human nature lies both the necessity of autonomy and the necessity of placing social limits on it.

PART II

the biological limits of autonomy

5

It's Only Human Nature

What is man, that thou art mindful of him? and the son
of man, that thou visitest him? For thou hast made him
a little lower than the angels, and hast crowned him with
glory and honor.

—Psalm VIII: 4–5

THE POLITICAL BRIEF for autonomy is a strong one: It gave birth to the
great democratic governments and institutions that ennoble us. Precisely
because autonomy is such an essential concept for a democratic culture
like ours, it is crucial that we understand it properly. To do so we must
go beyond a political analysis of *individualism* into a biological and psychological understanding of the *individual*. It will then be apparent that autonomy is but one of many unique biological conditions that must work in
concert to shape human conduct.

Both the possibility of autonomy and its necessary limits are rooted in
the human condition. By that we mean specifically human needs and
wants; the conduct people initiate to fulfill their hopes and to satisfy their
desires; and the interrelationships between the individual and the various
institutions necessary to support his survival. We must understand what it
means to be a human being and how different we are from all other animals.

When Genesis describes us as created "in the image of God" and when
the psalmist says we are "a little lower than the angels," they are celebrating
the uniqueness of our species. We are something special, a class unto
ourselves. Modern biology and psychology have only confirmed these great
insights of traditional belief.

Part of the problem in discussing human behavior is that, even today,
most people are abysmally ignorant as to how extraordinary and unique
is this species *Homo sapiens* (whose name comes from the Latin for "taste,"

85

suggesting good taste, wisdom, and sensibility; what other species "names" things?). Recently, it has become fashionable to condemn such concepts as arrogant "anthropocentrism" or, worse, as bigoted "speciesism"—as if looking at the world from other than a human perspective were either possible or desirable. We have been encouraged to think of ourselves as smarter chimpanzees or as "naked apes." These constructions are inaccurate and misleading. We are as unlike the chimpanzee, our nearest "cousin," as he is unlike the slug. We are as unlike other creatures as God—if God exists—is unlike us.

Most of us recognize the attributes that make human beings special. Our "autonomy," it will be seen, is one of these characteristics. What we do not always perceive is the relationship between those diverse elements. To honor any of the parts (such as autonomy) without recognizing the interdependence of those parts is to court disaster. We are now doing precisely that in our current culture, elevating "autonomy" over those conditions necessary to support it. Autonomy does not stand alone, and it will not guarantee a free society. Wrapped together in the movement for greater and greater autonomous rights, smuggled into the modern concept of individualism, are some dangerous and false assumptions about human nature.

Part II of this book aims to illuminate those special features of human nature germane to a critical analysis of modern American culture. It will become apparent that we are at a point where the political process—not God or nature—controls the future of our species. We must keep in mind the following points:

Human beings are born incomplete. The Talmud asks: "If God had intended us to be circumcised, why didn't He create us that way in the first place?" The answer given is that, alone among creatures, we are born incomplete, with the privilege of sharing with our Creator in our own design.

Human beings are obligate social animals. Human beings must live in groups if the species is to survive. For this reason we must at times constrain the individual to serve the common good. So argue the communitarians. Conversely, the individual is not pitted against the group in some monumental struggle since individuals and groups are inextricably—actually, biologically—linked. Libertarians, too, must respect this fact.

The human individual is shaped and realized only in terms of his relationship to others. The self is created in interaction with others and is, in great part, experienced through those interactions. Destroy the social structure, and you will inevitably damage the emergence of the interactive self on which much of what is unique and precious to humanity depends. A feral child—as those few documented cases have demonstrated—seems somewhat short of human. A severely neglected child will be limited in some of the most essential elements of humanness: compassion, unselfishness, guilt, shame, and conscience.

Human beings are born "free." By this statement we usually mean that they are unhampered by the genetic fixity that characterizes all other animals. This "freedom" is the root of the autonomy argument. Our capacity to be self-selecting is then elevated to represent that cherished concept called human freedom.

Human beings are also born with biological constraints and limits. These limits include a range of emotions, such as fear, shame, and guilt, that constrain antisocial behavior; a capacity for conscience; emotional directives toward caring for the helpless child; and other biological directives. All tend to rein in the unbridled "freedom" that would destroy a free society. The culture of autonomy fails to perceive these constraints as being as essential to human freedom as choice itself.

Biological limits to autonomy must be socially and culturally expressed. The biological limits to autonomy are not created hard-wired; they exist inchoate, in nascent form only. This is what T. H. White meant when he said in *The Once and Future King* that we are only "potential" in God's image. The limits must emerge in the course of human development. Their emergence depends on the presence of caring adults during the crucial stages of infancy and on societal values that encourage their emergence.

Human beings design and create their own cultures. Other animals live in and adapt to the environment that God or nature assigned to them. We do not merely adjust ourselves to our environments, we adapt our environments to ourselves. Indeed, we design our own. As it turns out, we are less-than-perfect designers. We currently live in a highly developed but flawed environment. We are not just victims of the natural world, we are capable of "victimizing" it. We respect autonomy, as well we should, but we ignore the conditions necessary to sustain it. We love it "not wisely but too well," and we may destroy it in that process. We can maximize autonomy only in an environment that also encourages pride, guilt, empathy, identification, love, duty, obligation, unselfishness, and hope. We do not currently live in such a society. Our present culture of autonomy, with its contempt for community, is critically close to a tilt point that will lead either to its destruction or a regression toward authoritarianism.

Thinkers throughout history have tried to define what is special about the human species, usually by examining one or another of those things we do that other animals do not. Both Aristotle and Hobbes emphasized language as our distinguishing feature; Marx, the capacity to invent and use tools; Aquinas, our capacity for reason; and Ovid, our upright posture.

Any such list is bound to be arbitrary, but certain distinctive human characteristics seem most pertinent to understanding our present confusion about human rights and responsibilities. The first is our freedom from instinctual fixation, without which none of the other characteristics would have significant influence over our conduct. The second is the culturally and socially regulated nature of human sexuality, which is relatively free from hormonal rhythms and reproductive needs. The third is our social mobility and variability, our freedom from environmental determinism, and our geographic and cultural diversity. The fourth characteristic is the human capacity for imaginative thinking and reasoning, the symbolic power that frees us from the limits of the here and the now. We do not just think better than other animals, we think differently.

BORN "FREE": BIOLOGICAL AUTONOMY

The one feature that is most central to our nature—to our very souls—is encompassed in our relative freedom from instinctual or genetic patterning, that is, in our biological autonomy. This feature speaks most directly to the primary concern of this book: how to motivate people to behave well, and how to change the behaviors of those who do not, particularly behaviors that are destructive to the self or the community. This "theoretical" concern involves a range of issues from the most mundane to the profound, from encouraging the use of seat belts and discouraging smoking, to decreasing drug abuse and increasing immunizations for poor children, to enhancing self-esteem, and punishing criminals. In all of these issues, our attitudes toward autonomy will influence our policy decisions. Only after acknowledging how free we are from instinct and genetic determination can we examine the limits of this freedom.

Human behavior is not rigid; it is largely free of patterning; it is flexible and adaptable. This unique aspect of our behavior, in all of its complexity, is the biological and psychological precondition for all those things we call freedom.

Human beings can survive without these fixed patterns because we can substitute intelligence to figure out solutions to problems that frustrate or threaten us. Thus, freedom depends upon our analytical ability to solve problems that would threaten the survival of lesser species. Historically, these biological facts were the determining factors in building the image of human beings as "rational" (quite different from intelligent or analytic) and self-determining creatures, different in kind from all other creatures.

And different—gloriously different—we are. The lives of most animals are completely and clearly determined by an intricate network of genetic commands that ensure their survival under the expected and traditional conditions of their environment. These animals are marvelous self-repro-ducing and self-replicating systems, geared for survival in the peculiar conditions of their environment, whether it is the frozen heights of the Himalayas or the dark recesses of the sea.

Most animals are like supercomputers programmed for their specific habitats. Therefore, they are only minimally adaptable. Change their envi-ronment even slightly, and they cannot survive. Some major animal forms, like the dinosaurs, have disappeared for all time. Most animal activities that seem imaginative, brilliant, and inventive are actually none of these. The organized behavior of insects is fixed by instinct, not by choice, and the stupid mechanical quality of such behavior will be revealed by the lethal persistence of such behavior in the face of changed environmental conditions that make the same behavior deadly. The giant panda will flourish with a plentiful supply of bamboo shoots, but it is bamboo shoots or nothing. The insect, whose behavior seems so efficient, so rational, so purposeful, cannot make even minor changes in that behavior to accommo-date a life-threatening change in the environment. This is the reason for the increasing number of endangered species as their habitats undergo human-induced changes.

Some species have managed to survive by the lucky emergence of a mutation that by the grace of God or nature can flourish under the new conditions. (The vast majority of mutations are deadly.) The thousands of varieties of closely related but independent species represent the mutations that survived under changing conditions of climate or food availability. Birds and beetles that appear indistinguishable to the amateur may actually be independent and different species.

The human being, in contrast, is a paragon of flexibility and adaptability. We are minimally programmed. Human behavior is dictated by very few genetic imperatives. Nature suggests, rather than commands, much that we do. Not only can we survive minor environmental changes, we seek out major ones. We migrated from the warmth of our African origins to the icy polar caps. We can live in grotesquely differing environments, changing our size, shape, and color without differentiating into different species. The Inuit and the equatorial Pygmy are not just kindred spirits but potential mates, unlike the arctic hare and tropical rabbits.

This freedom from instinctual patterning places a great burden on the developmental stages of the life cycle. The human being is born in a state of shocking dependency and remains so for a length of time unheard of in the animal kingdom. During this period of dependence, the individual's character and conduct must be molded and shaped. The moral human being will be either born or stillborn.

The great geneticist Theodosius Dobzhansky pointed out that, in developing culture, humankind has outstripped nature and found the "supra-genetic": "By changing what he knows about the world man changes the world that he knows; and by changing the world in which he lives man changes himself. Evolution need no longer be a destiny imposed from without; it may conceivably be controlled by man, in accordance with his wisdom and his values."[1]

Instead of changing our species to satisfy nature, we change our environments to serve ourselves. We build worlds out of our imagination and technologies that dazzle and bewilder members of our own species. When you have visited one beaver's hut, you have seen them all, wonderful though they may be. But with human architecture, each building is different. Moreover, beavers continue to build according to the same design and with the same materials as their primordial ancestor. The creatures at the depths of the seas occupy the same marine environment that they have for hundreds of thousands of years: constant, unchanged by any actions of marine species. But modern Londoners live in a world that could not have been imagined by their antecedents of only a thousand years before or even by their cousins the Yanomamö, who live in our own time. When we run out of arable land, we do not starve. We move to the arid and insufferable desert. We irrigate the land, and we air-condition the spaces we occupy. We create—God forgive us—Las Vegas.

We are blessed by our creator with the capacity to change our world, even our very selves. The conditions of human life are described with exquisite precision and awesome brevity in Genesis. God has endowed Adam and Eve with everything necessary for creature comfort. He has not endowed them with knowledge. They are free, however, and they are free to defy his injunction to avoid the fruit of the tree of knowledge. Our ultimate identity was shaped by their defiance. Before they performed that action, Adam and Eve were mysterious, inchoate, and hardly recognizable as human beings. Consider what happens after:

> And the eyes of them both were opened, and they knew they were naked; and they sewed fig leaves together, and made themselves girdles. And they heard the voice of the Lord God walking in the garden . . . and the man and his wife hid themselves from the presence of the Lord God. . . . And the Lord God called unto the man, and said unto him, "Where art thou?" And he said, "I heard Thy voice in the garden, and I was afraid, because I was naked; and I hid myself." And He said, "Who told thee that thou wast naked? Hast thou eaten of the tree, whereof I commanded thee that thou shouldest not eat?" And the man said, "The woman whom Thou gavest to be with me, she gave me of the tree, and I did eat."[2]

Now, here is a couple with whom we can identify. We know these inquiring, defiant, ambitious, inquisitive—and ultimately confused—people: the mother and father of us all. Ashamed, frightened, guilty, expecting punishment they know they deserve; whining, blaming each other—she did it, he did it, they did it, it wasn't I. We recognize the child that we once were and the child that remains within us always. It is not difficult to read the story of Adam and Eve as the story of development from the innocence of childhood to the guilt of adulthood—from dependence to responsibility. That may be one intended message of this complex tale that exists on multiple levels. At any level, the text is a story of the birth of morality.

Genesis describes the biological singularity of our species, the double birth of *Homo sapiens*. We are shaped by God in our potential and reshaped by human choice—by nature and by nurture. Each human being is constructed in such a way that as an infant it is born incomplete, awaiting the impact of the parent-controlled environment to determine whether it will develop into a fully mature human being or something less. This incompleteness explains the coexistence of Saint Francis and Adolf Hitler as members of the same species.

In selecting knowledge over safety, the primal pair, Adam and Eve, chose the risks and uncertainty of freedom over the security and restrictions of dependence. They thereby assumed responsibility for their own completion, becoming parents to themselves. They wove the capacity for good and evil into the fabric of human existence. There can be no moral creature without freedom and choice. A freedom that only allows one to choose well is no freedom at all. The concept of autonomy is epitomized in the story of the Garden.

Similarly, the emergence of emotional directives that limit our autonomy are here revealed as well. Out of Adam and Eve's defiance, shame, guilt, and fear emerge. These emotions constitute the stuff of which conscience will later be built. The moral human being—as well as the complex psychological human being that occupies the latter half of the twentieth century—is born, ironically, through the exercise of autonomy against the ultimate authority of God; we free ourselves from even the laws of nature. More precisely, with the birth of man, we redefine the rules.

There is nothing in lower animals equivalent to the freedom of will in the human being. Nothing can mitigate the command of animals' instinct. "Instinct," Kant has said, is "that voice of God that is obeyed by all animals."[3] By Kant's definition, the human being is not an animal, for we are constantly disobeying. This same notion is explicated with authority and elegance in Genesis. A generous Creator offers Adam the world, literally, with but one caveat: "Of every tree of the garden thou mayest freely eat; but of the Tree of the Knowledge of good and evil, thou shalt not eat of it."[4]

The primal pair disobeyed, and human beings were created anew in that disobedience. We continue to defy the call of instinct, often to our peril but also to our ennoblement. Perhaps the pivotal concept is not defiance but being true to our nature. In *Homo sapiens*, as in all animals, basic drives crucial for survival—thirst, hunger, the sexual drive—are genetically coded into the species. The power of the human design is so great that we are free to sacrifice or corrupt even life-sustaining activities. And we do so for purposes both noble and venal. With animals, activities that are necessary for survival are immutable.

Rousseau identified this essential difference in human nature when he stated that with the beast nature alone does *everything;* but with man he himself, as a free agent, cooperates with nature. The beast "chooses or rejects by instinct," and man "by an act of freedom." Moreover, "the beast cannot deviate from the rule that is prescribed to it even when it would be advantageous for it to do so, and a man deviates from it often to his detriment. . . . Nature commands every animal and a creature obeys. Man feels the same impetus but he realizes that he is free to acquiesce or resist."[5]

Or, to put it more simply, "an animal is at the end of a few weeks what he will be all of its life; and the species is at the end of a thousand years what it was the first year of that thousand."[6]

Having been freed from instinct, we are now free to design our world and in so doing share in the design of our very selves. To serve us in that purpose, we have the use of that extraordinary development of nature, the human mind, an essential adjunct to our freedom from instinctual fixity.

Reasoning and analytic abilities would be meaningless appendages without the freedom from instinctual fixity that alone allows us to use our intelligence to pursue our ends. Similarly, freedom would have no meaning without the kind of mind that can order the environment. Freedom of will has meaning only within the kind of thinking that is exclusively the function of the human brain, different in kind, not just in quantitative capacity, from that of all other animals. The kinds of choices that are available to lesser animals are trivial and insignificant. Such choices (Shall I eat the banana or the mango first?) can have only accidental significance for their individual survival and none for that of their species. No enlightened ape has ever discovered a means of manufacturing tools to enhance his struggle for survival against stronger predators. Only human beings are capable of making important decisions, and the survival of the human species will inevitably depend on them.

If the invention of the rifle and the plow demonstrates the vast chasm that separates the human being from his closest animal "relative," what can we say about the invention of the violin and the telescope! What bizarre "animal" expends the energy for such an abstract and nonutilitarian purpose as examining the stars? The building of the pyramids is in its complex way a metaphor for all that is singular in the activities of the human species. The purpose for which the pyramids were built is unrelated to individual or species survival. It is a testament rather to religious conviction, vanity, cruelty, wastefulness, aesthetics, imagination, and technology. In all of these aspects, the pyramids are characteristically and exclusively products of the human imagination. This opportunity for creativity, this opportunity for glory that is also an open invitation to disaster, is not available to other species. They must play it safe.

Animals are motivated exclusively by their individual and species needs as directed by their instincts. We are more often motivated by our dreams and aspirations. Food and sex and escape from predators dominate the actions and the "thoughts" of animals. But we are different. In any culture, beyond basic survival, behind many of our daily activities, people are motivated by symbolic aspects of existence—by status, fame, reputation, honor, and pride.

By contrast, other animal species are destroyed by chance, by catastrophes of nature, or often by the simple alteration of their environment, but never by elective behavior. No other animal will ever build an atom bomb. Nor will any animal consciously refuse food when it is plentiful and choose hunger for some long-range purpose. Overgrazing during a period of prolonged drought may destroy a species of cattle, but the cattle will be driven by their hunger to graze. No bovine Joseph will interpret the dreams of a bovine Pharaoh. There will be no rationing, no storage, no enduring of hunger in the presence of plenty, and therefore no eventual life-saving allocation in a period of want. Human beings are capable of anticipating a future different from the present, a future they have never experienced. When we desire to change human behavior, we must either seduce people with the rewards of a better future or deter them with the threat of a worse one.

HUMAN SEXUALITY: FREEDOM FROM REPRODUCTION

The other special features of human beings cannot be dealt with here in the same detail, but they must not be omitted from the portrait we are sketching. The second biological foundation of autonomy is the nature of human sexuality. Sexual reproduction and indeed sexual intercourse are obviously features we share with many lower forms of animals. However, human beings (together with the Bonobo, a close relative of the chimpanzee) are the only continuously sexed animal. Human beings have no mating season and no distinct estrus. The implications of this form of sexuality are profound. It is the foundation of romantic love and eroticism. In order to "get on" with other essential business of individual and species survival (gathering food, tending the young, avoiding the predator), we must place ritual—religious or cultural—limits on the sexual drive, since the seasons do not impose it. We must separate lust from love.

The sexual drive of the animal is automatic and unromantic. They just get on with it. Animals may be devoted partners, but although they may express biological fidelity and even monogamy (as with the goose) that puts human constancy to shame, they do not experience the romantic love that so influences human behavior.

Although we share sexuality with other animals, for human beings sexuality is different, not just in degree but in kind. One fascinating distinction is that we adopt self-imposed rules of sexual conduct. As in all animals, the human sexual drive is instinctually driven, but it is not controlled by instinct alone—we are free of instinctual rigidity. We impose social rules to govern our sexual behavior that, although they impinge on our autonomy, are also a product of it. Sexual mores, kinship rules, marriage, and the "rules" of sexual behavior are devices that emerged because we are free from genetic patterning.

If we were to adopt the casual mating habits of hippos or warthogs, we would not be "liberating" our sexuality, we would be demeaning it. When we adopt the casual mating of animals without their instinctual directives and limits—given the ongoing nature of human sexuality—we may well disrupt such social institutions as marriage, which serve to bind sexual desire to reproduction and child care. By destroying the conditions that support parenting, whether for economic or philosophical reasons, we would destroy the child—and not only the child, but the society that will later be shaped by those parentless children, will suffer. It is no coincidence, therefore, that the dissolution of the family today is occurring during a period when social rules are in flux and sexuality has been unhinged from binding commitments and relationships.

FREE-RANGE PEOPLE

Human beings are also the most wide-ranging of all animals. We cover distances unheard of by any other species and did so even prior to the advent of jet planes and ocean liners. We cross seas and climb mountains not "because they are there" but because we are inclined to venture forth into the unknown. And we have the capacity to adjust both ourselves and the environment to accommodate the natural world to our needs. We make a tool, we learn to use fire, and technology is off and running.

This wide range of ours, as well as our variability, ensured the continuation of a single widespread species. To survive in varied conditions—no other animal could—we design a variety of totally different cultures, each of which in its own way ensures survival in its environment. Especially in harsh and inhospitable environments, political and cultural constraints must then be designed to guarantee survival of the individual. Autonomy cannot be allowed to destroy these stabilizing factors, lest the culture, and the human beings dependent on it, be destroyed.

Today human beings as one species are slowly coming to share a highly interconnected global culture. Thanks to technologies of communication and transportation and to patterns of economic development, "mistakes" of a serious nature in one culture (particularly Western culture) will become universal. Before the expansion of Western culture, the variability of tribal mores, from the gentle Kung Bushmen to the aggressive Yanomamö, ensured that any self-destructive cultural values that might emerge would affect only the isolated tribe that dreamed them up. We are slowly becoming one tribe, with the same set of values. From the sere Sahara deserts to the wet rain forests of the Amazon, we all now drink beer and Cokes while watching the World Cup soccer matches on television or listening to Michael Jackson on tapes and CDs.

Directly related to our wide range is the fact that we are the most variable of all species, with the possible exception of those artificial species that are also a product of human technology—domesticated animals. We come in different sizes and different colors and different shapes—and despite all this variation we continue to breed true. We have not fragmented into various and multiple species. This very unity has led to the diversity that both enriches us and plagues us. Unhappily, human diversity has often been distorted by identifying an "us" and an alien "other," as though we were divided into different species, denying the glory of our species—that we are all one and the same even though we look different. If we all looked as alike as penguins, we would certainly have eliminated by now the racial bigotry that led to slavery and now a semipermanent underclass in America. On the other hand, perversely, our ingenuity would likely have found other sources of bias. Can anyone distinguish by naked appearance alone the Serb from the Croat; the Irish Catholic from the Irish Protestant; the Russian from the Chechen?

SYMBOLIC IMAGINATION: FREEDOM FROM THE HERE AND NOW

Beyond our reasoning powers is our imagination, our capacity for symbolic (conceptual) thought. The English biologist Julian Huxley observed: "Not merely has conceptual thought been evolved only in man; it could not have been evolved except in man."[7] Language (true speech), tool making (technology in its broadest sense), aesthetics, culture, and civilization are all products of this special quality of the special organ that is the human brain. Our capacity for anticipation and symbolization, so central to our motivations to do good and bad, are a product of this special brain and mind. Our capacity to anticipate reward and punishment, and futures we have not yet experienced, becomes a central feature in molding human beings. It is clearly a significant factor in making decisions. The results of our autonomous acts will vary drastically as we either encourage or discourage a capacity to visualize a future good that is promising enough to motivate us to abandon a present pleasure.

We should attend to the fate of the Irish elk: as Stephen Jay Gould has pointed out it has much to teach us.[8] This magnificent beast, during the course of its adaptation, developed progressively grander and more elaborate horns. Those males who had the largest horns won the battle of survival by attracting more females and by threatening their potential rivals. Eventually the Irish elk (ironically, neither Irish nor elk, but actually a deer) evolved such a massive ornamental headdress that it got caught on tree branches and could not flee from predators. Its former glory became the source of its downfall. What had originated as adaptive had become destructive.

At this stage, modern civilization is in many ways becoming like the horns of the elk. There are indications that the culture of autonomy has estranged us from certain necessary conditions of survival as human beings. Unaware, we may have passed the apex of adaptation and slipped onto the downward slope. What was formerly our glory and power—our love of freedom and the culture it has spawned—has now begun to reduce us. We feel increasingly impotent in the face of the rigid culture of autonomy that we ourselves have created and that now seems to control us.

6

Growing Up Good

Heaven lies about us in our infancy!
Shades of the prison-house begin to close
Upon the growing boy.
—WILLIAM WORDSWORTH,
"Ode. Intimations on Immortality from
Recollections of Early Childhood"

HAVING PAID OUR respects to the uniquely self-choosing capacity of human nature, we may now look at the less-than-lovely world we occupy and wonder how any self-choosing animal could have chosen this.

How can we have tolerated, let alone chosen, the disparity between the advantaged and the disadvantaged that exists in even the most liberal of societies? How can we have allowed the deterioration of safety and civility in the streets of even the most civilized of nations? Have we unwittingly encouraged it? Must we endure it?

We are interested in demonstrating how individuals—as citizens and as parents—can attempt to change certain socially destructive and self-defeating aspects of human behavior, and how and why we may have failed in the past. Although it is not easy to curb self-destructive and antisocial behavior, our biological nature itself can help us. The same nature that supplied us with autonomy also bestowed upon us attributes and mechanisms to check brute individual survival and to serve social unity.

We have built-in biological directives for altruism and social accommodation. These directives set limits to choice. Like most of human nature, they can be enhanced or destroyed by culture.

The prolonged period of dependence imposed on the human infant not only binds adults to the infant but gives them the opportunity to indoctrinate the child with values. Moreover, the conditions of reasonable care will allow the natural attributes for altruism and social accommodation to emerge naturally *without indoctrination*.

The social emotions of guilt, shame, and pride—uniquely human—are such powerful motivators, when they are present, that they can be exploited by parent and community to shape decency and moral conduct. They too are unfortunately also dependent on proper nurture. Even if the nurture is absent, however, we can still limit behavior by the use of fear, which seems to be relatively immune to cultural variability.

In the process of modifying behavior, we must understand what moves and motivates people. We must not act on the basis of some myth of human behavior that has been elaborated in order to sustain a specific political view of human beings. We must not, for example, overvalue rationality because we want to see ourselves as rational. "Education," whatever that means these days, is not the solution to every problem from AIDS to xenophobia.

The failure of Russian agriculture was its insistence on clinging to a discredited view of genetics. Mendelian genetics had proved that acquired characteristics are not inheritable, putting to an end Lamarck's theory, embraced by the leading Soviet biologist of the Stalinist period, T. D. Lysenko, that all kernels of corn are born equal, depending only on the nurturing environment to shape their final form. Lysenkoism, threatened by the obvious truth that what is genetically true for corn was most likely true for human beings, saw modern genetics as a threat to Marxist egalitarianism. By denying scientific data to preserve political mythology, the Stalinists managed to do a disservice to the complexities of both Marxism and science. Untold millions of people starved to death in the Soviet Union in defense of this mythology, aided in great part by collectivization enforced to serve a similar political purpose.

Of course, Mendel was right and Lamarck was wrong. Copernicus and Galileo knew whereof they spoke, despite the anxiety and arrogance of the Roman Catholic Church's hierarchy. We can defend the nobility of the human species without assuming that we are uninfluenced by genetics and without insisting that man must occupy the center of the universe. Similarly, we can defend the dignity of man without clinging to outmoded definitions of human autonomy and rationality.

We know that unlike any other creature, human beings are self-determining. We are obliged to do for ourselves basic things necessary for our survival that nature does for other creatures. We elect to be ruled by rulers, and we determine the degree of their power. Ants do not elect their queen and cannot choose to convert from an absolute monarchy to a constitutional monarchy or a democracy. The great apes live in primal hordes as they have from generation to generation. No feminist movement will emerge to alter these patriarchies. The hyena will live in a matriarchal society forever.

So apparent and so startling is this special quality of autonomy that it is tempting to exaggerate the degree to which we are self-determining, as well as to overvalue it. This exaggeration has led to the culture of autonomy that threatens our society to this day. We must now examine some real limits to our autonomy.

BIOLOGICAL LIMITS TO AUTONOMY

The freedom from genetic directives that partly defines human nature is not absolute. We have built-in biological constraints that limit our self-tinkering in order to help ensure species survival. Nature may not absolutely command us, but in certain areas crucial for survival it gives us more than just a small nudge in a vital direction. And it certainly sets boundaries.

Human beings can discover how to fly without wings, and we can penetrate the depths of the oceans without gills, but some things we cannot change. We obviously could not have survived as a species in a society that demanded permanent fasting or that interdicted sexual intercourse. Religions that made such demands would likely die out, unable to attract many followers given the powerful instinctual drives for food and sex that guarantee our survival. In addition, like most mutations, such religions would have been self-destructive. A totally homosexual society might have emerged, but without modern technology or vigorous recruitment, it could not have sustained itself. It has been hard enough for the Roman Catholic Church to maintain celibacy in the limited population of its ecclesiastical community.

Just as our individual survival demands nutrients, water, and oxygen, and just as our species survival demands sexual intercourse, our developmental nature "demands" certain cultural institutions that until recently were unquestioned. Foremost among them is a communal or family structure of some kind to support the human infant during its prolonged term of dependence.

Even before the rise of modern psychology, physicians were aware of an array of responses and automatic behaviors that act through neurological loops that bypass the brain, thus avoiding voluntary, conscious intention. These are the basic ("spinal") reflexes. They are not left to choice or chance. The sucking and clutching reflexes of the newborn demand no volition. They operate, necessarily so, in direct response to the appropriate stimulus.

Similarly, when a hand hits a flame, it is automatically withdrawn, without any analysis of the advantages or disadvantages of burnt digits. We have a whole range of such built-in autonomic and automatic patterns that are hedonically (pain/pleasure) controlled and reflexively driven to reinforce the possibilities of our survival. Even here, however, the human brain and will often have the capacity to override these life-sustaining, (basically) autonomic mechanisms. Take the simple spinal reflex of withdrawing a hand from heat; a teenage boy will test the limits of his "courage" by consciously overriding this basic reflex and enduring the pain to prove his "manhood."

In *Totem and Taboo*[1] Freud carried these observations one crucial step further. He strongly argued that certain *moral* behavior patterns—certain revulsions and attitudes—are as essential for the survival of the species (and the individual) as are these basic reflexes. They, too, he postulated, cannot be an accident of culture but must be built into the genetic nature of the species. Otherwise, human beings would not have survived for hundreds of thousands of years before they created culture or even discovered the facts of life that underlie many cultural institutions—such as the fact that sexuality and reproduction are related.

Most of the *emotional* responses that ensure the maintenance of the species relate to the conditions necessary to support the family and social life mandated by the prolonged helplessness of the human child. Incest taboos, Freud speculated, would be universal, because without them the social fabric of the family would be rent. Freud referred to many of these genetic directives as "instincts." Later psychologists substituted words like "needs" or "drives," recognizing the human capacity to override such directives, thus distinguishing them from mostly immutable animal instincts.

Similarly, much of sexual behavior is controlled and limited by strong and universal emotions that define a basic concept of privacy. Certain acts of modesty and shame around sexuality and body exposure seem never to be completely absent from any culture. The pudendal ("shameful") areas of the body are generally treated as private parts. This sense of modesty is essential in a species that is continuously sexual—that is, freed of estrus and mating periods—but is also biologically communal. Unlike other species, the human female desires and enjoys sex independent of her estrous cycle or even her life-period of fertility. This continuous sexual involvement encourages the strong male-female bonding—the foundation of monogamy and family—required to nurture and protect an infant so hopelessly helpless for such an exhausting length of time.

Some taboos are so deeply rooted in the emotional endowment of human beings that they are woven into almost every culture. Anthropology has supported the intuitive assumptions of Freud that incest taboos are universal. Nonetheless, the current stream of court cases and anecdotal accounts of incestuous acts reveal the capacity of the human being to perversely bypass biological warning signals.

Similarly, a loving and caring response to a helpless child must be present in order to ensure the protective and benevolent attitudes of the adult human being of both sexes. Child abuse cases, once again, only indicate how little is hard-wired in the human nature, whereas our universal revulsion toward child abusers testifies to a caring aspect rooted deeply in our psychological (and perhaps even genetic) makeup.

Even maternal protection of the young, which seems so natural, is a complex biological and cultural achievement. The first test of the new-born guppy is to escape from its mother, who views the baby guppy as an ideal postpartum feast. A guppy is born with this biological capacity and this genetic charge. The human infant is not. He is helpless and unable to protect himself in any way, so he needs maternal caring for his very survival—and better still, paternal caring as well. Adolf Portmann, the distinguished student of animal behavior, emphasized this dependence as the most striking aspect of human development, characterizing it as a "special extra-uterine first year."[2] Freud, too, would focus on biological dependence as the most profound influence on human nature and development.

Nonetheless, in the name of autonomy, the cultural institutions that we are creating erode even this caring for the dependent infant. The poverty and despair of ghetto life has combined with a sexual and moral revolution to produce the neglected child of the crack-addicted mother and the anonymous father.

Paternity—given the protracted nine-month delay between action (intercourse) and consequence (birth)—is less obvious than maternity; we know from certain tribal histories and other cultural data that paternity was not an early discovered phenomenon. However, a protective attitude toward the young must not be exclusively a "maternal" instinct. For otherwise the human father—physically stronger than the female of the species, like many other male animal parents—might see the newborn as a way to satisfy his primal appetite for food. Indeed, female tigers must protect their young from the very fathers that begot them. Some inherent protective response toward the infant must be presumed to explain why the human male, unlike the male tiger, does not view the young as a convenient comestible. Yet here too our culture of autonomy is demonstrating its capacity to destroy the communal bonds that sustain family life. We have reduced the distance between the man and the tiger.

Many other animals besides humans respond with a protective and caring attitude toward infantile creatures of their own kind. But to a dog in heat, one adult male is like any other (even one who happens to be her firstborn child). Not so with normal human beings: Our "young" are our young even when they are old.

In addition, the indulgence required for the human infant is enormous, considering how long that human infant is helpless and how incredibly helpless he is. The conditions of human dependence are enough to test the patience of a Job. A child will survive only with caring adults, and he himself will become a caring adult only if he is given attention and affection in addition to having his physical survival needs met. Attitudes that dominate adult human behavior, both social and antisocial, are formed during infancy. We must appreciate the role that dependence plays in moral development. Dependence allows us to set values. It allows for the emergence of conscience, it restrains selfishness, and it encourages beneficence. It is a period in which we shape future adult behavior, by shackling autonomy with internal moral constraints.

Only with this understanding can we appreciate how destructive has been the recent rise in teenage pregnancy and the demise of the family. Only armed with this insight can we build political support for policies to bolster the family or alternative structures of caring for newborns and young children.

Further compounding the problem is the fact that children reach a reproductive capacity at puberty, somewhere between the ages of thirteen and fifteen, but boys and girls of this age are totally incapable of assuming either the social or the economic role of parents or even of self-supporting adults. Through the demands of our modern technological society, we have extended the period of childhood well beyond its already extreme biological base. Allowing the current epidemic of teenage pregnancy to continue will not only bring more children into the world without adequate caretakers—a recipe for the social disaster we are already viewing—but will deprive the teenage mother of her rightful share of childhood and the education necessary for her entry into the middle class.

Further, if only the biological or survival needs of the human infant are met, with no caring or developmental support in the broader sense, the biological entity that survives may end up being less than human. A whole range of research now supports this supposition, starting with the pioneering work of John Bowlby on English children separated from their parents during World War II and that of René Spitz on institutionalized children.

Deprive a child of care in his formative years—as we do when we permit social conditions that destroy families but provide no alternative forms of socialization and caring—and he will repay us for this negligence with behavior controlled by neither love nor conscience. This "child" will roam the streets viewing other human beings in the way that a predator views his prey. This is the child who will father children without ever being a father. These aspects of his personality—and the economic disparities that encourage them—are the root causes of rape, spousal abuse, and child abuse.

In summary, nothing more clearly contradicts the individualistic assumptions of the culture of autonomy than the nature of birth and childhood. Social structures—community, family, state, and tribe—are not dispensable inventions of human history. The need for a social structure of some kind is a part of our biology and a necessary part of our development and survival; we could not survive as a species or develop true to type did we not have a social structure to support us. Social order is not something from which we can be "autonomous." Rather it is the precondition of autonomy. Autonomy theorists must certainly know this by now; nonetheless, they ignore it in their theories, and it is absent in the culture of autonomy.

A list of the biological limits of autonomy may be helpful at this point. These limits are not a group of independent elements; in human beings everything can act in concert with everything else.

The limits to autonomy are both internal and external. The internal limits include spinal reflexes; internal drives (hunger, thirst, libido, internal taboos and directives); incest aversion; care of infants; the primitive emotions of fear and rage, such as acting in a "blind rage;" and the social emotions (guilt, shame, pride, and conscience).

The external limits to the exercise of autonomy include appeals to rationality; appeals to conscience and the social emotions; and appeals to the primal emotion of fear (bringing us into the arena of coercion).

The complexity of human motivation is such that even coercive appeals to the emotions are filtered through a reasoning self that is free to say either "I'll take the pain for the reward" or "I'll be good—don't punish me."

All of the above limits to autonomy are understandable only in the context of the special nature of human development. A brief foray into human development will indicate how the social adult is "made." Just as important, it will direct us to the proper tools to reform or control those antisocial adults who will inevitably appear when we deprive children of the caring environment that is their birthright.

MORAL DEVELOPMENT

The typical response to danger in most animals is "fight or flight." The smaller the animal, the less likely it is that it will be capable of surviving by fighting, so flight—or escape—is the primary mechanism of survival. Fear is "contagious" in many animals, and a mother's fear, when transmitted to the young, initiates a flight response in the young—muscles are tensed, blood pressure is elevated, hormones are released—mobilizing it to flee the predator. Think of the frenzied flight of a herd of gazelles at the scent or sight of marauding lions.

However, the human infant is capable of neither flight nor fight. Survival for this helpless creature has never been possible in these terms. His first method of survival is neither to fight nor to flee but something akin to clutching or clinging. The primitive grasping mechanism of the newborn is a genetic imperative to cling to the supporting parent.

It is impossible, of course, to establish directly the thinking of an infant. Most authorities agree that the earliest stage of infant consciousness is dominated by the child's sensations, not yet necessarily even emotions. He senses his needs through the pain and discomfort of hunger, wetness, pinpricks, chafing, and so on. The newborn does not "feel hungry"; he experiences the pains and pangs of hunger. He screams (is this rage or reflex?), and seemingly his scream produces a warm suffusion of liquid into the gastrointestinal tract, relieving the distress. The child is not aware of the complicated sequence of events that transpires between the outcry and the blessed alleviation of pain. How can he possibly know that his cry awakened his somnolent father, who then nudged his somnolent mother, who then went through the detailed business of warming a bottle or preparing for nursing?

At this early age, it must be presumed, the infant may feel that the cry *itself* produces the satisfaction of desire, creating a false sense of power. Only gradually will the child become aware of the environment around him as an alien or other entity, and with this awareness his concept of himself and his relationship to this environment will change radically and forever.

With the realization that there are things (out there) that are not part of himself, the child not only becomes aware that he is not magically omnipotent, he also becomes aware of his own helplessness. In a fall whose psychic proportions must rival the fall of the angels (perhaps the inspiration for that myth), the child is reduced in his own perception from the highest of creatures to the lowest—helpless and vulnerable.

What can keep the child from sinking into despair or total panic? (Some psychoanalysts have actually postulated such states.) The child is saved from despondency by the recognition of the presence of other figures in that environment who are strong and capable. The groundwork has now been set for acceptance and fear of authority and, conversely, for the potential coercive powers of authority over the individual.

At every stage of this scenario, the child undergoes a profound alteration in his sense of self and the relationship of the self to the "community," which at first is only the caring parents. With adequate caretakers the normal child will then enter a stage of peace and security. The process of building trust, bonding, and socialization will be initiated. Without caring, the child's survival will be rooted only in a hostile and distrusting self.

With time, the normal child learns what may be the most crucial lesson in modifying human behavior and conduct. He learns that these parental figures have the power not only to give pleasure and support needs but to withhold and punish. The child then realizes that parental protection comes with conditions. His parents' willingness to serve his needs is related to the nature of their relationship with him and their feelings for him. And their approval is related to his conduct.

Character traits in children emerge through a pragmatic trial- and-error method, particularly in early childhood stages, when moral attitudes are being implanted. The child does wrong, and he sees disappointment, chagrin, hurt, or anger on his parent's face. He does right, and he sees pride and love shining down on him. That strange and long dependence period of the human animal is the crucible in which adult behavior will be shaped and through which "free will" will be constricted or redefined.

The typical child, like an amoeba, will most likely test the environment randomly in all directions until she locates a behavior that works to achieve what she wants. Because the human child does not forage for food, her only important survival activity is securing the approval of the parents who will nurture and sustain her. The child will try all means to ingratiate herself with the parents and gain their love. If charm and wiles work, she will use them. If those means are disdained but obedience and order work, they will become her devices of choice. Children are masters at reading their parents' moods. They have to be. Their lives—at least, as they see the issue—depend on it. In this way, personality and character are formed. For example, if ingratiation and charm never work, if one's parents are moved only by performance, the child is well on the way to becoming a workaholic—or in defiance, a dropout.

If this trial-and-error method, generally called *conditioning*, were the only way we learned behavior, our learning would be contingent on the totality of our experiences (and the generalizations we draw from them) over the course of our lifetime. This is simply not the case, however: we learn to behave in other ways that are independent of specific conditioning or even specific life experiences. Well before he acquires language, the child is learning. He learns by multiple methods that have little to do with parental education or teaching in the accepted sense of the words.

Modeling, and the related phenomenon of *identification,* operates in ways quite independent of conditioning. A child will consciously model her actions after her parents', thereby absorbing whole integrated patterns of behavior that are determined by the parents' past conditioning (or modeling) rather than her own. The child thus learns wholesale—through bulk purchasing, if you will—whole chunks of unexamined perceptions and behaviors that will be integrated and absorbed into the self and then become determinants of her future actions. Such modeling explains why children infuriatingly seem to absorb some of our worst traits, even while we are lecturing them to do otherwise.

Beyond modeling, which is often conscious, an unconscious identification with the parents occurs. The child swallows up the images of his parents (through the process of *introjection,* as psychoanalysts call it), and those images become integrated into his self-image. These idealized parents become a model against which the child judges his own behavior. When he finds himself wanting, he feels that sense of self-betrayal called guilt. This is why guilt is such an internalized emotion.

These two devices, modeling and identification, one conscious and the other unconscious, explain why children tend to become like their parents rather than like other people's parents, and rather than what their parents ideally want them to become. Identification is so powerful a process that it mystifies parents who do not appreciate the distinction between their instructions and their actions. A child who has only confusing or negative models will be forced to adopt the traits of those only available models, or else—like the psychopath—will seem to have no standards, no sense of right and wrong.

In the absence of parental models, a child is forced to depend exclusively on his own trial-and-error experience for learning—often in the context of a hostile and unsupportive environment. His sense of identity will be impoverished, his insecurities will be enlarged, and his view of life will be shaped by models of brute survival. He will overvalue fear and intimidation; he will rarely become sensitized to empathy and compassion. He will still hunger for some enlarged sense of self, some heroic figures to emulate; and he will still seek the comfort and security of community. If the only symbol of power is the local drug dealer, he will emulate him. If the only source of community is the street gang, he will find community there.

It is heartbreaking to observe this process happening in our culture, when we know that the presence of an active and caring adult could serve as a constructive and positive model for children's acculturation. Our failure to intervene—to supply caring figures who will serve as models—impoverishes the individual and threatens social order. For this reason the establishment of early childhood day care centers—universally available, mandated in conditions of proven parental neglect—should be a primary political goal. Close behind should be locally run but nationally supported outreach and community programs that provide older children and adolescents with the sense of community they need in a safe but peer-oriented and flexible environment. Moreover, economic development and job training programs for adolescents and young adults must be revitalized and expanded, even in times of low national unemployment and prosperity, because we cannot afford the permanent exclusion of a sizable segment of our young people from the legitimate economy.

In summary, the prolonged period of human dependence allows parents sufficient time to actively mold the child into their model of a proper adult, to instill moral values and principles of proper behavior. The unpredictable results of these efforts are apparent to anyone who has raised a child. Still, our children are our products, for better or worse, and we shape them to our conscious or unconscious designs. But for children without loving caretakers, who will be the models? Who will set their standards? Who will define their constraints? And what kind of lessons will those children be learning about the world they are about to occupy and about the rules necessary to survive in that world?

By the time the average child reaches adulthood, he carries within him certain values and sensibilities that force much of his behavior into automatic patterns. In other words, he has been so indoctrinated by the conditions of his early childhood and by the values of his caretakers that his in-built set of values and propriety, his conscience, and his self-image impose limitations on his freedom of action.

Parents continue to modify their children's behavior during their formative years, through love or neglect, thereby further shaping attitudes. Attitudes and behaviors that are set early in life will seem to have the fixity of instinct. Toilet attitudes and concepts of modesty are only two kinds of behavior that are formulated early and that are dreadfully difficult to change, but there are many other fixed patterns of behavior. Feeding patterns are notoriously culture-bound and are set early. It is the rare American who can eat a dog or rat with gusto, even though these are delicacies in other cultures.

MANNERS AND CHARACTER

Early childhood modeling has its most noticeable effects in two areas that seem vastly different: the first, manners and mien, the second, character and values. Manners and mien are expressed in apparently unimportant behaviors—forms of dress, social conduct—the "superficial" behaviors that distinguish one country or one period from another. Character and values, by contrast, control the most profound aspects of our behavior. They determine whether and under what circumstances we will sacrifice our self-interest, or even our self, on behalf of others or in the service of ideals that transcend survival.

Manners is the word that was traditionally used to describe the socially correct way of acting; polite behavior or etiquette. The term now has a quaint and old-fashioned ring to it, which is a significant statement about the changing relationship between the individual and the community today. Instilled in young children, manners make for an automatic behavior, often inexplicable to those children who practice them once they are grown. Thus manners represent a limit on autonomy as self-choosing behavior. Ambrose Bierce defined *habit*, in his *Devil's Dictionary*, as "a shackle for the free."[3]

At one time, children "instinctively" rose when an adult entered the room. They may have had no idea what purpose was served by this behavior, but they would rise in the same way that a yo-yo rises when it is tugged. With maturation, many would recognize the reasoning behind the behavior: it was a sign of courtesy or attention, an act of respect, an acknowledgment of the status of the other person, and perhaps an offer of services, such as making a seat available.

Although rational reasons underlie some conventions, for other conventions the reasons have disappeared, and manners have become merely a preservation of form over substance. Men were once instructed from childhood to walk on the outside of the sidewalk when accompanying a woman, long after the era of mud roads and rambunctious horses was past, although now thieves ride by on motorcycles to grab purses. For some men, it became a mechanical and meaningless behavior. One of the advantages of social conventions of this sort is that, addressed as they are to unimportant situations, they free us from having to analyze each and every situation and allow us to concentrate on decision making that is more important.

Rules are important, but they are not fundamental. Rules, like laws, explicate acceptable and unacceptable behavior that is not generally negotiable. They make life simpler; they allow a child to identify right and wrong without having to become an analytic philosopher. We do not want children to have to stop and consider every piece of behavior in order to decide when self-interest should be abandoned in the service of love and generosity. Automatic and unconscious compliance with the common morals at the most primitive level is the first goal.

One justification for good "manners," then, is that they constitute a guide to decorum for the undramatic aspects of everyday life. They allow for the mechanization of certain behaviors—so that one can concentrate on more complicated problems. Like an experienced driver who automatically maneuvers through traffic, she is free to concentrate her rational analysis on more difficult issues, such as the wisest route to avoid traffic at this time of day, rather than on when to release the clutch or turn on her direction signal indicator.

Manners also make life easier for those who must share a common space. They can count on one another's predictable behavior: they won't urinate on the front porch; they won't grab food from each other's plates; they won't steal from someone else's purse when she temporarily leaves the room. Manners once dictated positive behavior as well as constraints. There was a time when one could depend on deference to the elderly, courtesy in common public intercourse, and decency in public language.

Manners are one substitute for instincts or instinctive behavior. That they are sometimes concerned with trivial aspects of life does not mean they do not add elegance to life in general. They express courtesy and respect. There was a more civilized, somewhat more gracious quality in the days when an adolescent boy would automatically rise to offer a seat in a train or trolley to an older woman or, for that matter, to an older man.

Manners contribute to civility by defining, logically or otherwise, a public behavior to which we all are expected to conform. In that sense, they are far from trivial. They define a code of conduct that pays homage to the public space and acknowledges a limiting force on self-indulgence and impulse. Manners carried within them a set of values and expressed a concern for decorum and decency. Manners were an attempt to maintain a distinction between "civilized" and "uncivilized" behavior.

The deprived and disaffected develop their own standards of behavior. Shaped by a different set of experiences, they adopt a different set of "manners" that advertise a different experience. Different codes of conduct will be instilled in a child by a neglecting and brutalized early environment, like "every man for himself"; "dog eat dog"; "it's a jungle out there"; "it's them or us"; "only the tough survive." Power, not attachments, is the source of survival. Obscenities or even signatures scrawled on the common walls of public spaces announce the graffitist's elevation of the "I" over the "us." This phenomenon is understandable but is still a warning of danger.

The romanticizing of graffiti as art by Norman Mailer and other members of an indulgent liberal community is baffling and may even be dangerous.[4] It legitimates a clear violation of and contempt for community. The graffitist is simply expressing that which he has been taught. What is the rationale of his defenders? Graffiti is an act of narcissistic defiance; a sign of contempt for the common space. Urinating and defecating on the public streets are its logical extensions. They too, incredibly, now have their defenders.

Although the automatic dimensions of social behavior limit autonomy, human behavior is still free, for better or worse, of the rigid fixity of insect behavior. Humans can reinvent themselves with incredible rapidity. In one generation we can reverse the social habits of centuries. We see it in every so-called social revolution, whether it is the sexual revolution of the 1960s or the technological revolution still in progress.

Behavior that is directly related to moral values and conscience is more resistant to change than manners and is more important to social order. Behavior that is linked to survival is usually less flexible and less culture-conditioned than either moral behavior or manners, for it reinforces a biological and genetic directive. The almost reflexive readiness of most parents to risk their own survival recklessly and willfully to save the life of their dependent child is but one extreme example. For most of us, such behaviors are automatic, so dovetailed into our intuitive responses that they seem immutable. However, even this fundamental biological human trait is capable of erosion via cultural assault. We assume that it is the genetic nature of human beings to behave in this "normal" way, and we are shocked and bewildered when we discover those among our kind who violate such patterns with "unnatural" acts of child abuse.

The power of improper early conditioning to dissipate our human potential is incalculable. Those distorted few who abuse their children violate the biological directive on which the future of our species is built: the compassionate concern for the dependent child.

What of the adolescent who can calmly hit a fellow human being over the head with a lead pipe to gain the contents of a purse? The absence of any constraining guilt or shame in his behavior implies a defective conscience mechanism *that is unlikely to be reparable*. When a conscience-free individual emerges because of an inadequate or corrupting early environment, no amount of goodwill, understanding, compassion, or, for that matter, psychotherapy is likely to rectify the problem. Stripped of the higher social emotions that characterize our species—guilt, shame, pride, and conscience—such persons are governed only by the more primal emotions that we share with other animals—fear and rage. Self-control in these individuals will reside in fear of retribution, not in remorse.

It is essential to recognize that lessons learned in childhood persist in the unconscious of every adult. This being so, it is simple logic to recognize that adult behavior can be influenced as readily by appeals or threats directed to the unconscious as by overt threats in everyday life. The teenager, for example, does not even acknowledge the possibility of his death. Threats of exclusion from his group and the contempt of his peers are normally more powerful sources of motivation for him and therefore are more coercive in shaping his behavior than any adult warnings about the risks he and his peers are taking. One example is in the use of condoms in this age of AIDS. Statistics have shown a particular reluctance to use condoms among teenage Latinos, for whom paternity and potency are linked; condoms seem to threaten the *machismo* so respected in their culture. Peer counseling has generally proved more effective than adult counseling in getting sexually active teenagers to use condoms.

By the time the average child reaches adulthood, she carries within her certain values and sensibilities that will drive much of her behavior into automatic patterns. In other words, a set of constraints and imperatives will be imposed on her freedom of action by an in-built set of values operating both consciously and unconsciously through the mediation and collaboration of her conscience, her identity, and her self-image. It goes without saying that a lack of conscience and constraints is as influential as their presence in shaping conduct.

The crucial fact that must be kept in mind when considering early "education" or reform is the enormous plasticity that exists in early life— and *only* in early life. In changing people's behavior, age is a lever that becomes progressively shorter. At birth a newborn child is all potential, awaiting and demanding the modeling of a behavior pattern; the arm of the lever is extraordinarily long. With a proper fulcrum and a proper position, Archimedes said, he could move the world. The parent has that fulcrum and that position, but most particularly in the first few years of life. This knowledge demands that we emphasize a prophylactic rather than a therapeutic approach to antisocial behavior.

Although it is always possible to alter some of the automatic reflexive behaviors that are patterned during our developing years, it is usually extremely difficult. These instinct-like patterns of human behavior, once they have become ingrained, are stubbornly resistant to change, as our dismal experience in attempting to rehabilitate sexual offenders demonstrates. But we need not reach so far from normalcy to find examples of failure in rehabilitation. Think of overeating and smoking; think of physical cowardice or reckless abandon. The amount of money that has been wasted on misguided efforts at rehabilitation, after the damage has been done, is heartbreaking compared with what those efforts could have accomplished during the pliant period of infancy. Research findings supporting this observation have been demonstrated over and over again in a multitude of disciplines.

All of the complex factors of the human condition influence our significant choices. Those choices are rarely purely rational or totally functions of external stimuli. Behavior is influenced by forces in operation *within* the individual, forces both biologically and developmentally determined, as well as by what is occurring in the external world.

However, conscience mechanisms are not either wholly present or wholly absent. The world is not inhabited exclusively by saints and sinners. All of us are driven by those elementary needs for survival, increasingly interpreted in terms of relative power. Middle-class Americans struggle not for food and warmth but for those symbols of status and power that are equated with survival in the metaphoric world in which they live and strive. All of us are tempted by money and its privileges. All of us want security, and we will often define it at ludicrous levels of comfort. The disparity between the rich and the poor in our society is testament to how ready the righteous majority are to violate their professed ideals for the sake of personal gratification and symbols of worth.

Most of us need some social constraints to support even reasonably well-developed consciences. Does anyone doubt that the fear of imprisonment for violating the tax code supports honest reporting of income? Those who doubt it need only compare the rate of tax cheating in a country like Italy, where serious penalties, until recently, had not been imposed, with the rate in the United States. Visualize any law that constrains social behavior—without its punitive conditions. Imagine laws against stealing, graft, embezzlement, income-tax evasion, stock manipulations, gambling, fraud—all nice white-collar crimes—without serious punishments, and speculate how the decent middle-American white "law-abiding" citizen would behave. Or simply think of those crimes where punishment is minimal or rarely enforced—speeding, for example—and see how many people violate the law. The rich use their political influence to ensure that loopholes are built into tax legislation to protect their interests. But how many of the rich would forgo these special tax provisions and pay more taxes out of a sense of fairness, equity, or social justice?

Beyond the limitations of conscience, other influences drive us to destructive behavior, often self-destructive behavior. Patterning and addiction are powerful forces constraining autonomy and rational choice. Rational persuasion almost never works with addictions. The addict knows only too well that he would be better off not overeating, drinking, smoking, or using drugs.

Consider cigarette smoking. By now everybody knows about its health effects, but in some people the power of the addiction overcomes the knowledge of harm. If, however, a smoker loses a lung because of lung cancer, her *terror* of death will reinforce her knowledge and in all probability assist her in giving up the addiction. The one group of people that are most likely to find little difficulty in giving up smoking are those who have had a lung removed due to lung cancer. Emotional appeals have proven to be essential in disrupting addictive behaviors.

Conscience mechanisms also differ in structure and strength. We are all likely to behave most selfishly when we feel threatened. The pull of survival is immensely strong, and insecurity is likely to enhance our sense of vulnerability. A diminished ego will allow a person to perceive the smallest slight and reduction of status as a threat to survival. Unfortunately, as far as pride and self-respect are concerned, we live in a world of the poor, the maimed, the halt, and the blind. Modern society seems to conspire to make us all feel inadequate in one way or another. Insecurity can drive even reasonably decent people to abandon their standards of decorum and responsibility and into the dominion of fear, rage, and irrationality. The formations of armed militia throughout the rural areas of our country are only one part of the growing population of the insecure. Insecurity carried to its extreme becomes paranoia.

We do not have to look to the lunatic fringe for evidence of paranoia. Such perverse irrationality is evident in the crazy behavior of human beings in their automobiles when they risk life and limb to answer the "disrespect" and humiliation of being "cut off," as though the phrase were being applied literally. More evidence is present in the tragic corruptibility of seemingly honorable people when presented with the power opportunities of political office. Greed, selfishness, or ambition can overcome a sense of fairness and honor, unless the latter is reinforced by fear of punishment.

Conduct is always determined by a balance between the limited conscience of an individual and his selfish passions. This being the case, even with the best of people, a certain amount of persuasion and coercion is necessary to ensure a socially acceptable environment. We must recognize that most human beings are more likely to respond to emotional forces—intimidation, compulsion, coercion, shame, pride, threat, or reward—than to appeals to reason. Even in the mature and responsible adult, knowing good often does not result in doing good.

Good conduct will always require emotional reinforcement, whether it be via the social emotions of shame, guilt, and pride or the primitive emotion of fear. If we wish to campaign against drunken driving, cigarette smoking, littering, and the like, education is never enough. If we wish to campaign for safe sex, avoidance of drugs, protection of public spaces, respect for the law—education is surely not enough. Education must be reinforced by appeals to the emotions. Advertising executives know this, and it is time for social scientists, philosophers, policymakers, and social leaders to acknowledge it as well.

We are not as free and self-determining as we would like to believe, and we are not as independent as we pretend to be. We must face the fact that we are not as rational as we would like to think we are. The rational roots of our conduct are pathetically overvalued. We must appreciate the power of emotions over human behavior in order to effectively institute changes in that behavior. Despite a preference in the culture of autonomy for rational persuasion and a bias against manipulation and coercion, persuasion rarely works. It is coercion on which society must depend.

7

Irrational Man

Whatever the Moralists may say about it, human understanding owes much to the Passions, which by common agreement also owe much to it. It is by their activity that our reason is perfected. . . . The Passions in turn derive their origin from our needs and their progress from our knowledge.

—JEAN-JACQUES ROUSSEAU, *Discourse on the Origin and Foundations of Inequality among Men*

KNOWING GOOD AND DOING GOOD

The philosopher William Barrett said: "The centuries-long evolution of human reason is one of man's greatest triumphs, but it is still in process, still incomplete, still to be. . . . The rationalism of the Enlightenment will have to recognize that at the very heart of its light there is also a darkness."[1] Rooted firmly in human freedom from instinctual fixation and in the human capacity for rational analysis is the fallacious assumption that *Homo sapiens* is the rational animal. We must do some uprooting of this notion in order to get on with the political and social work before us.

The problem with this assumption is twofold. First, people are not as self-directing as they think; and second, people are not as rationally driven as they believe. In other words, we are not the autonomous animals we like to think we are. Nor are we the self-directed creatures we pretend to be. To know the good does not ensure that we will do the good.

Certainly, human beings possess an unparalleled capacity for analytic and synthetic reasoning. We can analyze complex problems, understand the implications of diverse behaviors for our future well-being, and appreciate the consequences of not behaving rationally—and still we do not always behave intelligently or properly.

119

Saint Paul said: "I do not understand my own actions. For I do not do what I want, but I do the very thing I hate. . . . I can will what is right, but I cannot do it."[2] Saint Paul knew whereof he spoke. The ability to reason is not the same as the ability to behave reasonably. We all know that we should eat more sensibly; lose weight; stop smoking; exercise regularly; practice safe sex; tell the truth; spend less and save more; call our parents regularly. We all know what is good, or good for us, yet like Saint Paul, we do not do that which we know.

Still, in the minds of most of us the implicit assumption persists that a considerable—if not an absolute—relationship between knowing good and doing good must exist. Hasn't the Western philosophical tradition, beginning with Socrates, reassured us that moral knowledge will lead, by a straight (if not a short) route, to just moral conduct? This misconception about the effectiveness of rationality in directing behavior has cost us considerably. It is an error in understanding human psychology. The culture of autonomy compounds the error with its ethical assumption that somehow education is morally superior to appeals to emotions.

As a result of this assumption, the first response to every social problem these days is to appoint a commission to study it. The next step is to recommend some expensive program involving better *education* about the problem in question, be it AIDS, drunken driving, or drug abuse. The final step is to spend billions of dollars on useless programs in areas that demand effective solutions.

Not a day goes by without evidence of our persistent adherence to the myth of rationality—and of the price we pay for it. Consider the following from the *New York Times*: "Despite an educational effort in South Carolina, women are not taking a B vitamin that can prevent one of the most common and devastating birth defects, a new study shows. Experts say the finding bodes ill for less intense national efforts by groups like the March of Dimes to persuade women to take folic acid and raises a more general question: what does it take to get Americans to change their health habits?"[3] What, indeed. If a woman will not swallow a simple vitamin pill to protect the child *in utero*, will she give up alcohol, smoking, or drugs—much more difficult behavioral adjustments? Yet in deference to an ideal of autonomy, Americans persist in their faith that they can "educate" away the behavior that is destroying children, vulgarizing public spaces, and diminishing private lives.

Our society seems prepared to endure massive pain and injustice—the spread of AIDS to children, a burgeoning population of the homeless, avoidable illnesses—in order to protect our illusions about human conduct. Understanding human motivation is no longer an academic exercise but is essential for effective public policy and for the social survival dependent on the programs established by it.

It isn't as though common sense and everyday experience have not revealed to all of us how irrationally we are prepared to behave. Each of us surely can recall incidents in our own experience that raise doubts about the assumption that knowledge informs conduct. How is it that we so readily deny in our public policy that which we have experienced in our personal lives?

Twenty-some years ago, during a conference with what were then the leading lights in moral philosophy, a number of unpleasant incidents arose and were called to the attention of the organizing directors of the meeting. One of the distinguished philosophers, a married middle-aged man, was sexually involved with an undergraduate who was working for him. Another distinguished philosopher managed to use this conference (and subsequent ones) as an occasion for sexual pursuits aggressive enough to be labeled harassment by current standards.

Beyond these sexual misdemeanors, our moralists demonstrated a degree of hostility, a lack of spiritual and emotional generosity, a level of personal calumny and gossip-mongering, and a proclivity for both backbiting and public humiliation of their colleagues that were, charitably speaking, at least equal to the prevailing academic norms in medicine, law, and the social sciences. At the same time, we are all acquainted with relatively unsophisticated individuals—people who would not know a utilitarian from an electrician or a deontologist from an endodontist—who often act with grace and goodwill and lead generally moral existences.

Over the years, anyone involved in the academic world must come to the inescapable conclusion that philosophers—despite their considerably greater knowledge of ethics—comport themselves by no higher set of moral standards than nonphilosophers. One is therefore reluctantly driven to recognize that a direct quantitative relationship between knowing good and doing good does not exist.

Knowledge will influence behavior only in that person who *wills* the good and is committed to pursuing it. This kind of behavioral change through knowledge has come to be called, since the onset of the feminist movement, consciousness-raising. It is a potent force for changing behavior. If a man has done something that unwittingly shames, humiliates, or hurts a woman—and if he has a conscience and a desire to be fair and kind— then when he becomes convinced that his behavior unwittingly produced these results, he will change his behavior.

Saint Paul, with all his problems, thus represents the easy case. Paul is a man of values, who despairs of being capable of always behaving in ways that support his values. Paul *wants* to do the right thing and has a clear definition of some concept of the right. He has values we can respect. He suffers guilt and shame when he falls short of his ideals, and these emotions motivate him to do good. He has a conscience. And still he often does wrong. Unaccompanied by this good will, knowledge alone will never change behavior.

LESSONS FROM PSYCHOLOGY

Any attempts by society to modify individual behavior must always keep in mind the two most important insights of Freudian psychology. First, we live in the world of our own perception. Second, we are not always aware of our own motivations.

It does not matter if we are smart, successful, rich, and beautiful; if we think we are not, we behave as though we are not. The slights we feel may be only of our imagination, but the agonies that follow from them are as real as the pains from malignancy. A person blessed with abundance may see himself as deprived. A man deprived may perceive himself as blessed.

The multitude of choices that most of us make in our daily lives do not involve our biological survival but serve instead the often artificial symbols of power or respect that are equated with cultural survival. What motivates most people these days is not the stuff of survival but the symbols of power and status. The money that corrupts is used not for the purchase of porridge, woolens, or shelter. The street gangs that tyrannize our inner-city schools are doing so for eighteen-carat gold chains, $200 Nikes, and other "necessities" of their life. The status symbols for which they kill are no different in principle from those that motivate the embezzler and the Wall Street manipulator.

Freud offered an explanation as to why we behave less rationally than we would like to. Much of our behavior, he said, is a product of feelings and perceptions of which we are unaware. Most of the behavior that we consider rational is actually motivated by unconscious needs and then, after the fact, supported by a logical rationalization.

Given these facts of life, efforts at changing behavior must be directed at the unconscious perception as well as the conscious biases of individuals. Appeals to reason alone will not suffice. The contribution of irrational elements to determining behavior, long recognized by psychiatrists and psychologists but ignored or resisted by many theorists of autonomy and many policymakers, must now be acknowledged.

It is not that policymakers do not already implicitly understand the role that fear, for example, plays in conforming conduct. They do. Every time legislators pass a law (and a threat of punishment)—whether it is a law against smoking in certain spaces or against sexual harassment—they are acknowledging that knowledge and self-control have failed or are inadequate to our purposes. When we pass a law, we add fear of punishment to the process of reasoning, acknowledging the need for social controls to supplement self-control. This awareness of the limits of personal self-control, this understanding that social controls may enlist emotional appeals, must be extended into many areas beyond law that serve the individual and the public good.

Anyone who walks the mean and dirty streets of our mean and dirty cities today is more likely to meet Attila the Hun than Saint Paul. Who are these people who seem to have no proper values? What are we to do with those who do not conform their behavior to proper social standards because they do not accept them? What of those with no shame or guilt, with no pride, no models—or worse, with negative models? How do we change these people? We would like to make them want and choose to do and be good; but the conditions that make it difficult or impossible for them to do so, as we discussed, were decided early in life. We must be prepared to settle for the less ambitious goal of simply getting them to behave well whether they wish to or not.

In modern times the most concerted challenge to the concept of autonomy has emerged from the field of psychology, not from philosophy. By observing the irrational and therefore self-defeating aspects of much behavior, psychologists have questioned how voluntary, how freely chosen, such behavior is.

In the field of psychology, autonomy has no backers. The two major influences here, behaviorism and psychoanalysis, may be antagonistic in every other way, but they are traditionally joined in embracing a form of modified determinism. Both see behavior as a complex endpoint, the result of forces and counterforces (or accretions of conditioning) accumulated over the years, patterning the individual in such a way as to produce an inevitable result. In other words, the psychologists, without necessarily realizing what they were doing, have reaffirmed some kinship between the human being and the ant, substituting psychic determinism for genetic determinism.

The image of man that emerged, particularly in B. F. Skinner's *Beyond Freedom and Dignity*,[4] is of a man chained to the past by a series of conditioning experiences that force him into predictable patterned responses. Skinner abandons freedom altogether—he denies its existence. It is a myth that human beings perpetuate about themselves, he says, in order to assert their superiority to the lower creatures, to whom Skinner would link humans in a simple continuum. Like the Grand Inquisitor, he urges us to abandon freedom for survival and happiness. For Skinner, this choice is not a major dilemma, because freedom is but an illusion.

Psychoanalysis, on the other hand, was dragged kicking and screaming to a semideterministic view of human behavior with which it has never been quite comfortable. Psychoanalysts continually struggle to visualize a self-governing and responsible human being, while constantly revealing new ways by which present behavior is hemmed in and structured by past events. Their struggle has been a curious one. The heart of psychoanalysis has been with freedom, whereas its discoveries constantly challenge autonomy. In the end, psychoanalysis significantly eroded the Enlightenment image of an independent, autonomous, and rational human being.

Freud postulated that human choice is constricted by the sense of reality that each child constructs out of his early childhood experiences. His developmental past, his life experiences, will shape the way he interprets the present as an adult and will therefore predispose him to a limited number of choices. The pivotal biological fact that shapes human conduct, Freud concluded, was the state of dependence, which we have previously discussed.[5]

Humans' freedom from instinctual fixity is, therefore, mitigated by cultural rules, internalized perceptions, and constraints imposed by socialization. Values will be fixed, and the emotions to support them will be developed, that will influence all future behavior. The individual may still be perceived as "free," but his choices will be constricted by his developmental history.

Some children grow up with such guilt over lying that each attempt to lie will produce an agonizing dilemma, even when their lying serves a beneficent purpose. Others will see lying as their only survival mechanism in a harsh and punishing environment. Both will tell the truth at times, and both will lie, but their predictable responses will differ vastly.

In summary, the basic conditions that influence adult conduct are set early in life by our parents and our culture. They are shaped by a confluence of factors: parental encouragement, coercion, conditioning, emotional intimidation, identification, and all of the other familiar devices that parents employ—consciously or unconsciously, calculatedly or unwittingly—to convert their children into good boys and girls. These diverse elements will shape the character, personality, ideals, values, and conscience mechanisms that become the adult framework through which reason or influence must operate to change behavior.

For some of us, reason will lend a capacity to step back from ourselves, understand that which is driving us, and then take conscious control of our actions in accordance with our goals or values. But it will do so only in some people and only in limited circumstances. For the most part, individuals will respond to everyday events reflexively based on their past experience, or they will respond to key emotions that transcend mere logic or judgment by triggering certain patterned perceptions and sensibilities. All of them may lie or break the law at times. To some it will come easily, and to others only with pain.

EMOTION ALLIED WITH REASON

Feelings are too often represented as the opposite of rationality: either you behave emotionally or you behave reasonably. If this were the case, then human beings, with their extraordinary rationality, would need *fewer* emotions than other animals. In actuality, we have a repertoire of emotions unequaled in the animal kingdom. Why?

Fine-tuned feelings are not the antagonists of reason; they are the necessary by-products of reason. Because we are intelligent creatures, we are freed from instinctive and patterned behavior to an unparalleled degree, and we must make difficult and important choices constantly throughout our daily activities. We must also make relatively unimportant decisions.

The need to analyze each and every decision before action would paralyze or severely diminish our day-to-day functioning and could even threaten our survival. Therefore built-in mechanisms to automate human behavior are a part of our biological heritage. Our emotions guide us to quick action.

Some of these reflex patterns are akin to those in lower animals. Like other animals, human beings possess certain "instinctive" responses to danger, tendencies to fight or flight. Sensory perceptions of pain force us to withdraw our hand from the hot pan, without requiring the brain to carefully analyze the desired action.

Beyond these basic survival tools, however, is a repertoire of special attributes that human beings alone possess. Among these uniquely human features is a wide range of emotions that are "unnecessary" in lower animals. These we will call the *social emotions*. In a small mammal like a mole, where almost everything essential to the survival of the individual and the species is programmed in (mating behavior, food-gathering, care of the young, flight from predators), the only emotions necessary are those that direct the physiology to prepare for either fight or flight, fear or rage.

The long-range and subtle decisions made by the human animal— whose actions must often be decided upon by analyzing, thinking, and planning as distinguished from making predetermined and hard-wired responses—require the assistance of emotions that can, in simpler cases, bypass that analysis. Guilt, shame, and pride will mandate certain behavior without our having to analyze the pros and cons of the various options. Feelings guide us in the exercise of choice.

PHYSICAL SENSATIONS AND THE PRIMITIVE EMOTIONS

Sensations of pain and pleasure are common mediators of survival in the lower animals. Humans are not immune to these hedonic controls. We avoid pain and seek pleasure, as is evident in the effectiveness of rewards and punishments even in our sophisticated culture. Still, even here we are different. The human brain, with its multiple functions of examining, evaluating, and controlling behavior, can allow us to steel ourselves to the pain of the physician's needle without withdrawing our arm—or even to defy the torturer to protect our comrades or our cause. These are examples where human rationality can overcome even the reflexive responses that normally bypass cerebral judgment.

In the complex world of the human response, people often endure pain for a higher rational purpose. They endure present pain for later good, or they pursue an unselfish action that brings pride or joy, even though it involves self-inflicted pain. Through their perceptual capacity to weave a past and future into a blueprint for the present, they know that some pain is worth enduring for higher values, future pleasure, or pride of service. This endurance is not, however, the inevitable consequence of the interplay between feelings and cognition.

Pain, however, is still not fear; it is not an emotion. Pain requires intimate physical contact. By the time the jaws of the tiger are at your throat and you feel the pain, the perception of danger does you little good. What you need to enhance your survival is a way to *anticipate* the tiger's arrival. This occurs in evolution with the emergence of modalities known as distance receptors. *Distance receptors* are the organs of smelling, hearing, and seeing, and in some animals the sense of vibration. These distance receptors allow an animal to locate—before physical contact—that which is about to destroy it. Distance receptors make possible physical anticipation—which is a long way from the intellectual anticipation of human beings but is still a remarkable increment in the struggle for survival. Anticipation buys time.

Anticipation of imminent danger produces the emotions of fear and rage that humans share with lower animals. These primitive emotions induce action and produce the bodily changes for that action. They alert the animal to fight or flight and they even indicate which is appropriate. They are motivators at the most primitive level of survival. Human beings too have an emergency system built on fear and rage that is a basic part of our physiology. When the Paleolithic predator stalked us, we ran—and we still may. However, as human beings, with our capacities for learning and for symbol formation, we can go well beyond the signals of our distance receptors.

THE SOCIAL EMOTIONS

If human beings possessed only these primitive emotions, they would be forced to design societies that control behavior only through the exercise of fear. Tyrannical despots have created just such societies, and they continue to do so to the very present. Fortunately, the stability of these societies is limited. We aspire to more—and we are capable of more. We are capable of conforming human behavior to social needs without reducing people to the level of frightened and survival-driven animals.

Consider the "bizarre" behavior of soldiers in wartime. It is a far cry from the programmed behavior of insects in battle. Some potential soldiers become conscientious objectors. Soldiers facing battle could run, but that would be "cowardly," a concept that is specifically human. We are endowed with a whole range of conflicting emotions, like shame and pride, which counter our natural "instinct" to run from danger and avoid death. We will not run, even though our bodies are straining to do so, if it would make us seem cowardly. *The Red Badge of Courage* by Stephen Crane is an almost clinical study of the interplay of fear, shame, and self-respect.[6]

The daily newspapers of our metropolitan centers display the perversion of self-respect when young people seek respect not from the moral agents of the community but from the street gang that has filled the vacuum left by an uncaring culture. Here self-respect can be challenged by a stare—a sign of disrespect—and answered with a gun.

Even if human beings had only the emotions of fear and rage, however, they would still behave differently from most other animals. Our imagination, a super-distance receptor, and our synthetic reasoning permit us to anticipate threats even during periods of maximum security and comfort: to prepare in the best of times for the worst; to recognize that there are seasons, that the balm and plenty of summer will inevitably give way to the cold sparseness of winter. Because of our intelligence and imagination, we need not see the first frost before we have stored the harvest.

We do not endure pain simply to enhance our personal survival. Altruism still does motivate behavior in many of us. At rare times it may even call for the risk or sacrifice of individual life to support the group on which all individual survival depends. It is a natural part of our biology. But it must be encouraged by social attitudes and nurtured by our social institutions.

Because human beings often experience conflicting messages—"save yourself" versus "women and children first"—behavior directed to group survival over individual survival must be reinforced by emotions equally powerful and countervalent to the primary survival emotions of fear and rage. The social emotions of shame, guilt, and pride serve this purpose. We must learn how to encourage their development in each individual, and how to use or even manipulate them to serve the social good on which the good life, if not mere survival, depends.

In the culture of autonomy, the social emotions have not fared well. Self-mastery and critical detachment should be the hallmarks of the autonomous self. However, the "self" that is emerging in this self-involved culture of ours is an isolated self. Here the emphasis is on "fulfilling," "experiencing," "expressing," and "being true to" one's self. This emphasis omits that the self is most fully realized in relationships and within a culture that encourages a readiness for commitment and involvement.

The extension of an individualistic philosophy that idealizes "doing your own thing" and "letting it all hang out" has proved to be devastating. With the indulgence and relativism of modern social attitudes, the community shame that might have discouraged antisocial behavior is being replaced by a subtle encouragement of it. Graffiti is an art form; the criminal is a victim; the gang leader is a community organizer; gay bathhouses are a cultural aspect of a unique lifestyle; the homeless woman living off the streets adds diversity to our local landscape; the athlete who flouts the law is a macho hero; the Wall Street manipulator who arbitrages money to bring down the stability of economies is a financial genius. Ultimately we will have to change the culture of autonomy if we are to change individual behavior. Our society cannot afford to create an atmosphere in which going to prison is a badge of honor rather than a mark of shame.

There has been a general tendency, in this age of "self-actualization," to liberate people from the emotions of guilt and shame—as if they have no purpose other than to punish us. But guilt and shame are the noblest emotions, those that specifically define the human being as "a little lower than the angels." And they are essential to the maintenance of civilized society.

These feelings most profoundly shape our personhood and are most central to being human. They are vital for the development of the most refined and elegant qualities of human potential—generosity, service, self-sacrifice, unselfishness, love, and duty. They support our ability to feel remorse. It is for this reason that we focus on those few emotions—guilt and shame and their other half, pride. They are the building blocks of that magnificent self-regulator that is known as a conscience, the core of the moral animal.

We must live in social groups, and the social emotions encourage social living by providing internal, self-imposed restraints. Building internal constraints on behavior minimizes the need for external ones, thus allowing for a *freer* society and *freer* individuals. A proper understanding of the social emotions is essential in order to maintain the liberal society. In a social structure that minimizes shame and guilt, however, we are forced to utilize fear and external controls to stabilize society. We will be compelled increasingly to resort to fear of punishment—the one emotion that persists in even the most uncivilized of human beings. It should be obvious that a culture that minimizes the need to feel guilty or ashamed, that liberates people from moral standards that restrict their drives will inevitably require a more controlling and restrictive—a more fear-oriented—social structure. It should be obvious, but it has not been so. It is time for a revival of guilt and shame.

GUILT

It is safe to assume that everyone reading this book has felt fear. However, we cannot make that assumption about shame or guilt; some people never experience these feelings. They are not, however, the fortunate ones, and we are not fortunate to have them in our midst. A failure to feel guilt is a basic character flaw. It is the hallmark of the psychopath or antisocial person, who is quite capable of committing the vilest crimes without feeling any emotion of guilt. What, then, is guilt? What will distinguish it from related feelings?

If one were to ask a group of people to recall a situation in which they recently felt guilt, it is likely that at least half would describe something else—guilty fear. The qualities that characterize guilty fear fall into the caught-in-the-act or the about-to-be-caught category. We all know that panicky feeling when we are in the process of an immoral, illegal, or disapproved action and we feel the hot breath of authority on our neck. That rush of sickening feeling that we are about to be apprehended and punished is not guilt—rather, it is guilty fear. The primary emotion is fear. It is *guilty* fear, because it is fear that is clearly related to some wrongdoing that we acknowledge.

If you are casually driving at sixty-five miles per hour (when you know that fifty-five is the local limit) and suddenly hear the unmistakable sound of a police siren, then glimpse a highway patrol car in your rearview mirror, that fluttery feeling through your chest is guilty fear. Here guilt is only the modifier; *guilty* is the adjective to describe the kind of fear you feel.

The emotion you feel is not the product of having been bad but of having been *caught* at being bad.

Suppose now that as you apprehensively watch the approaching police car, it passes you by to flag down a car that whizzed past you only moments before. What do you feel? If it is relief, the emotion you experienced at the first sound of the siren was guilty fear. If you were disappointed at not receiving a ticket, then what you felt was true guilt.

The distinguishing test between the two is the relationship of the feeling to exposure and punishment. When guilty fear alone is present, getting away with an immoral or illegal action brings immediate relief and delight. Guilt, however, *wants* exposure. It needs exposure because it needs expiation and forgiveness. The most profound and immediate relief for this feeling is to confront the individual who has been offended or harmed by the action and who is capable of relieving the feeling of guilt.

Guilty fear, then, is relieved when the threat of exposure and punishment disappears, whereas true guilt often seeks and embraces exposure and punishment. Guilty fear is "us against them," "them" usually being the forces of authority. Guilt, on the other hand, represents the noblest and most painful of struggles; it is a battle between us and ourselves. Guilt is mitigated or alleviated only by acts of expiation. The purging power of the confessional, so clearly recognized by the Roman Catholic Church, acknowledges the central role of guilt, both in Christian theology and in everyday life.

We must not constantly rationalize the behavior of the antisocial. We can understand it, in order to be compassionate or to control it, but we must not romanticize it. Society and morality are best served not when people feel *less* guilty when they do wrong, but when they feel guiltier. One would think that someone versed in Christian theology would understand this insight best. Yet when one young man, hours after hammering his ex-lover until her head "burst open like a ripe watermelon," consulted a priest who barely knew him, the priest almost immediately advised him to put away his guilt and begin the process of "forgiving himself."[7]

The result of an increasing population of people "free" of guilt will inevitably be a more restrictive and harsher society. Lacking inner constraints and with appeals to guilt or pride ineffective, society will be forced to depend on fear, the only controlling emotion left, to support order. In our current political environment the calls for harsher and harsher penalties for criminals represents just such a development.

It is obvious that guilt is a different order of emotion from fear. Fear and rage are emotions oriented to the survival of the organism. They served as the primary protective devices for the individual in the primitive world of predator and prey, and in the days before law and civilization. What survival purposes are served by feelings like guilt, love, and caring? Would we not survive more adequately if unencumbered by such sentiments—if we greedily fought for each scrap of food even to the point of personal gluttony even as our weaker neighbor starved? We would not.

Remember that community is a biological necessity for the individual human being. Guilt forces us to abandon selfishness and the immediate fulfillment of self-interest. By forcing us to heed the needs and pains of others, guilt binds us to those whom we need for our own survival. Our seemingly unselfish acts serve our selves in ways that are not always apparent in our everyday battles for survival.

Above, beyond, and serving survival, guilt is a guardian of our goodness. It is an internal judgment that forces us to endure pain in order to do good. "Guilt becomes a way of putting oneself before a sort of invisible tribunal which measures the offense, pronounces the condemnation and inflicts the punishment," Paul Ricoeur has said.[8] We have judged ourselves and been found wanting. The feeling of guilt is thus seen as the pain of self-disappointment. It is the anguish we experience when we have not lived up to our standards of how we ought to behave and what we ought to be. We have somehow or other betrayed some internal ideal self. The intense pain of that anguish—and more important, the anticipation of that pain—powerfully motivates those people who can experience guilt to conform their behavior to their ideals rather than to their impulsive desires. You may covet your neighbor's property, but you will not steal it. Guilt not only serves species survival; it ensures that the species warrants survival.

SHAME

Shame is a sister emotion to guilt. Both serve the same purposes, facilitating the socially acceptable behavior required for group living. Neither is primarily devoted to personal pleasure. Both deal with transgressions against codes of conduct. As such they are devoted to the values and survival of the group in opposition to the selfish interests of the individual. They are supporting pillars of the social structure. Their purposes are the same, but their modes of action differ.

Guilt is a more internalized and personal emotion than shame. Its you-against-you orientation allows no buffer and no villain except yourself. The emotion of shame, by contrast, is primarily communal. Guilt is almost exclusively an inner-directed emotion, whereas shame incorporates the community, the group, the other directly into the feelings. This is why Aristotle, in defining shame, focused on it as a pain in regard to "bad things . . . which seem likely to involve us in discredit."[9] Aristotle described shame as the feeling that involves things that are disgraceful to ourselves or to those we care for.

"Bad things," "misdeeds," "discredit," "disgrace"—all these words reflect the elements that define shame, which entails both a misdeed and its exposure. Shame requires an audience—if not realistically, then symbolically. Shame is fear of a public exhibition of wrongdoing, of being exposed in front of a group. Guilt often drives us to seek exposure, but shame begs for privacy. Again, Aristotle recognized this when he said: "Shame is a mental picture of disgrace in which we shrink from the disgrace itself and *not* from its consequences."[10]

Of course, while we seek to hide in an attempt to avoid exposure, the punishment of shame continues. We will constantly act as though we are about to be exposed, and we will crave inclusion in the respectful presence of the group. Therefore, without necessarily revealing the source of our shame, we may, like Jean Valjean in Victor Hugo's *Les Misérables*, devote our energies to the reestablishment of our social standing; we may strive for reconciliation. Acts of social good are often efforts to reenter the society from which our shame has driven us.

In that masterpiece writing on shame, *The Scarlet Letter*, Nathaniel Hawthorne succinctly captured the public agony of shame. Hester Prynne is an accused and convicted adulteress. As her punishment, she must wear the scarlet letter A so that she may be publicly recognized and her crime publicly acknowledged:

> Continually, and in a thousand other ways, did she feel the innumerable throbs of anguish that had been so cunningly contrived for her

by the undying, the ever-active sentence of the Puritan tribunal. . . .
When strangers looked curiously at the scarlet letter—and none
ever failed to do so—they branded it afresh into Hester's soul. . . .
From first to last, in short, Hester Prynne had always this dreadful
agony in feeling a human eye upon the token; the spot never grew
callous; it seemed, on the contrary, to grow more sensitive with
daily torture.[11]

Shame tends to encourage behavior that binds the comfort and good
of the individual to the community's survival. It also allows the community
to join in the enforcement of moral behavior, rather than leaving this up
to individual responsibility and internalized models. The shame and disgrace of imprisonment, a form of punishment seen as most humane by our
society, is important in controlling those parts of the population that are
capable of feeling shame. White-collar and middle-class criminals should
serve some prison time, even if it serves no rehabilitative purpose. Imprisonment is an announcement of a violation of community standards, and the
shame is part of the punishment.

All of this presupposes the presence of a community with which the
individual can identify and to whose standards he can conform. It must
be a moral community. But what is happening today? If the only community
available is a street gang, then the "socializing" emotion of shame will
likely drive its members to conform to the perverse standards of the gang,
in which arrest and imprisonment, rape, and even murder may be badges
of honor rather than symbols of shame. In the gang, being soft—compassionate—earns contempt. To romanticize the gang as "at least some community" that the neglected adolescent can join is dangerously wrongheaded.
It ignores the moral purpose of community.

When the controlling power of shame is undermined by the destruction
of community pride or by the alienation of the individual from any sense of
community, antisocial behavior is facilitated. One example seems prophetic
and paradigmatic. In the summer of 1977 the city of New York suffered
a total blackout, extending in most areas for over twelve hours. Secondary
to the blackout, a rampage of looting and arson occurred that shocked the
entire community. In the immediate aftermath, in an exceedingly sensitive
and prescient editorial, the *Amsterdam News*, a leading Harlem newspaper,
acknowledged as one of the key forces in that riot the failure of leadership

to supply ideals, to support values, and to bind the group of individuals into a community.

The television interviews were more telling. One adolescent described the riot as "the best day of my life, like Christmas with everything free." When asked whether he felt there was anything wrong in looting, his answer was extraordinarily revealing. "The police couldn't do anything," he said, "because everybody was doing it, even 'old women and pregnant ladies.' "

In his perception—whether true or not—we see the undermining of the major forces for social responsibility. "The police couldn't do anything," therefore there was no guilty fear. "Everybody was doing it," therefore whatever guilt may have been felt was mitigated by the sense that looting was a communal standard of behavior. And no shame of public exposure may be feared when even "old ladies and pregnant women," those two most hallowed symbols of propriety and goodness—the matriarch and the Madonna—support the activity.

The breakdown of moral community and the absence of shame and guilt as mechanisms of social control are pervasive in society today and are by no means restricted to the poor and the inner city. What is one to make of the behavior of executives in the cigarette industry, who were willing to hide the evidence of their own researchers and disseminate their toxic products to their fellow human beings? And what of their cohorts in crime, the advertising executives who utilized their creative gifts to spot weaknesses in vulnerable populations, adolescent girls and boys, and to seduce them into a fatal addiction? It is not difficult to recognize the deficiencies in the lifestyle of the neglected ghetto child, but how did the conscience mechanisms of the privileged in our society become so attenuated?

Somehow the corruption of individualism reaches out into the affluent suburbs as well as into the inner cities. Certainly the competitive winning-is-everything psychology with which most boys in our culture have been raised has played its part. For them, losing and failure are the greatest disgrace, well beyond selfishness and venality.[12] A heartbreaking case study of the corruption of a middle-class boy by a middle-class institution may be found in Gary Alan Fine's study of Little League baseball.[13] The game that was presumed to teach sportsmanship ended up teaching that winning is all. This disappointing observation is apparently still valid. In 2001 the

New York City team was disqualified and its Little League World Series title taken away because its star player was overage and that fact had been hidden from Little League officials.

PRIDE

Human social behavior is driven not only by the aversive force of painful emotions like guilt and shame. There is a positive reinforcement that encourages us to sacrifice our selfish needs for a common good. Life, for the human being, is more than the avoidance of danger. We are also reward seekers. And unlike the lesser creatures, the beasts of the field, the rewards we seek are not just the nutrients that support our individual biological survival.

We are created as aspirers. Ovid, in his beautiful metaphor, tied our upright posture to our questing nature: "And, though all other animals are prone, and fix their gaze upon the earth, He gave man an uplifted face and bade him stand erect and turn his eyes to heaven."[14] We crave achievement, mastery, and purpose because they extend the meaning of human survival beyond the mere perpetuation of the biological shell. There is a unique experience of pleasure in performance, and in doing good, that is in its way the ultimate driving force for noble behavior. That pleasure is the experience of pride.

Although the experience of pride is evident early in childhood, it too must be nurtured into proper channels. The development of innate tendencies will be either encouraged or discouraged depending on the responses that early expressions of pride elicit from parents. A child's actions are influenced by parental attitudes so subtle, so artfully and unconsciously signaled and received, as to create the impression that the actions are "innate" and not taught.

This interplay between child and parent is a potent factor in the way a child learns to distinguish between good and bad in his early random behavior. When he does something, he almost invariably looks to his mother for approval or disapproval. That *looking to the mother* is surely an organic part of the adaptive process. Even if the appeal for approval is answered only with a smile or a perfunctory "I'm looking" or "That's lovely," a response is required. Someone must be there! Someone who shows care must attend the developing child. In those who are offered the proper cues, externally reinforced pride will eventually become internalized. We will continue throughout life to feel pride in terms of the good things we produce and the good things we do—in our productions and in our performance.

Internal pride is an essential ingredient of maturation. It is our incentive, and at the same time our reward, for abandoning the pleasures of dependence. Pride is the pleasure in achievement that supports independence. It is an added incentive to abandon the pleasures of childhood for the more elusive gratifications of maturity. Pride, then, like guilt and shame, is an emotion basic to the survival apparatus of the thinking and social animal that is the human being. In any society the sources of pride must be monitored. If the game of pride is played out only in terms of money, we will produce boardroom swindlers and inside traders. When the game of pride is played out in terms of terror and turf, we will have street gangs.

The weakness of the social emotions is that although the potential for them exists in all humankind, their emergence and maturation—unlike the primitive emotions of fear and rage, which are culture resistant—must be encouraged during childhood. Guilt, shame, and pride can operate only when they have been seared into the operating mechanism of the self. They presuppose the existence of a better inner self, of an ego ideal, a conscience. And their existence is dependent on caring parents—or reasonable surrogates—nurturing the inchoate self during the early dependence period with proper values and supplying adequate models of comportment. Someone must be there to instill and define those standards—those moral values.

CONSCIENCE

To repeat: guilt, shame, and pride are all present in potential form in the newborn child, but unlike the brute emotions of fear and rage, they demand a proper environment for their full flowering in adult life. Nature supplies that potential; nurture must elicit it. The mechanism that will mediate these uniquely human attributes and create that semidivine creature, the human being, is conscience.

Freud struggled with the idea of conscience, later to be labeled the superego, all of his creative life. His first foray led to the idea of an internalized and punitive parent we carry around with us in our unconscious. In this early view the individual continues to operate in selfish pursuit of instinctual and primitive pleasure, controlled only by his fear of punishment.

According to this view of conscience, we behave well because, whether the parent is actually present or not, we assume him to be lurking within us. Like some omniscient Peeping Tom, he sees all and is prepared to punish all. Conscience, in this view, is simply a mechanism to avoid punishment or rejection. Even this limited view would place human beings a cut above the beast. Anticipation, imagination, and conceptual thinking are all essential to the workings of the internalized parent.

Surely conscience represents more than mere constraint. If it did not, the human being would not be much different from the domesticated dog. Freud, recognizing this, evolved a richer concept of conscience in his study *Group Psychology and the Analysis of the Ego*.[15] Here he stated that each individual contains within her self an internalized image of an ideal self—an ego-ideal—by which the person judges her own behavior. We respond with pride when our behavior conforms to our ego ideal, and we respond with humiliation, shame, and guilt when we fail that better self. This ego ideal represents the powerful motivating force of guilt, shame, and pride. Guilt is not fear of the other, nor fear of punishment: it is not fear at all. It is our painful disappointment in being less than we want to be.

Now we have a new view of behavior and emotion. We're not driven exclusively by selfishness, the id, or instincts of survival, constrained only by fear. Not all instances of kindness and charity are simply approval-gaining mechanisms (although many may have started that way). Good behavior becomes a part of our sense of who we are and who we wish to be; it is an integral part of our interactive self.

When the conscience mechanism is in full play, it is a leading instrument in controlling human behavior. However, deficiencies and lacunae in the conscience allow people to act without the moral constraint imposed by intense and painful feelings of guilt and shame and loss of self-respect. Only the constraints of conscience and the feelings—guilt, shame, and pride—that mediate it can control the basic selfish "instincts" for survival, which are fear, rage, greed, and envy.

Once in place, the social emotions—particularly shame—can be used to coerce behavior in adult life. When a thug threatens you, he draws on your fear of anticipated pain. When a blackmailer threatens you with exposure, he draws on your sense of shame. Imprisonment is both a threat that is feared for its own sake and a source of social shaming. In at least a few instances the state uses shame legitimately to change behavior, such as by publishing the names of scofflaws or men soliciting prostitutes.

Guilt, as distinguished from shame, is most effectively utilized by groups other than the community at large or the state. It is the weapon of choice within the family—and not just with infants. The elderly parent's sighs of unspoken chastisement, often in an attempt to coerce the son or daughter into a specific behavior, are as effective as overt demands. A plaintive, elliptical comment is often more effective than a direct demand, because it cannot be explicitly countered. "It's been so long since your father has had a chance to chat with you," translates as, Come to dinner Sunday. Or "Your poor brother, if only he had your opportunities," translates as, Why don't you lend that unfortunate child some money? These tactics and enjoinders have given guilt a bad name. They are devices consciously used to force behavior. On the other hand, the behavior being forced may in itself be both reasonable and good. And the very guilt that may now seem coercive was once a cornerstone of character-building.

PART III

the ethical limits
of autonomy and
the uses of coercion

8

The Multiple Meanings of Coercion

"That's a great deal to make one word mean," Alice said
in a thoughtful tone.
"When I make a word do a lot of work like that," said
Humpty Dumpty, "I always pay it extra."
—LEWIS CARROLL, *Through the Looking Glass*

ORDINARY DEFINITIONS OF *coercion* have the advantage, as well as the
drawback, of binding it closely to autonomy. In common usage, coercion
is something that takes the authorship of an action away from the person
doing it. The will originating the action and the intention are not one's
own, but someone (or something) else's. In contract and tort law, *coercion*,
duress, and *undue influence* may be used by defendants to counter liability.
Coercion may make an otherwise legal agreement null and void. When
you are coerced into signing a contract, it becomes invalid, because it is
recognized that your signature does not represent your legally binding
promise or agreement.

The same sense of coercion as the negation of autonomy is found in
Black's Law Dictionary, which says that it "may be actual, direct, or positive,
as where physical force is used to compel an act against one's will, or implied,
legal or constructive, as where one party is constrained by subjugation to
the other to do what his free will would refuse."[1]

The word *coercion* comes from the Latin *coercere*, meaning "to surround,"
and even more suggestively from two older Latin words, *arca* ("box" or
"coffin") and *arcere* ("to shut in"). To coerce is to contract the space of
free movement and action around a person, making the space of self-
sovereignty and self-mastery smaller and tighter. Autonomy is the opposite—expansive and enlarging. In this common usage, autonomy and

coercion are defined by each other's absence: one is autonomous if one is not coerced, and to the extent that one is coerced, one is not autonomous.

The flaw in this common definition is that it inevitably casts coercion in a bad light. For many people, no matter how practically significant it may be, coercion is never *ethically* respectable. In certain conditions it may be necessary, therefore warranted, but it is never completely approved.

In addition, the term *coercion* has been extended to include almost every conceivable external influence on behavior, and they have all been pronounced bad. The culture of autonomy respects only the freely chosen act of the individual, an act that by implication has been chosen through rational analysis of all options. That is not the way people behave. To understand coercion, we must have some awareness of motivation from a psychological perspective.

MOTIVATION

Freud's version of human behavior has permeated modern dynamic psychology, and his basic theses, if not his language, have been absorbed into everyday lay sensibility. It will serve our purpose to use this understanding, which views behavior as dynamic, developmental, and purposive (or motivated). This view of human behavior may be summarized as follows:

All behavior—excluding simple spinal reflexes—is the complex result of a number of forces and counterforces that operate on the individual at the moment of action. Some of these influences arise from the past, some from the present; some work on us unconsciously, some are actively chosen. All of them will operate in concert to lead to some specific conduct: to run from the mugger or attack him; to stop smoking or rationalize about it; to practice safe sex or, just this one time, take a chance. These multiple forces constitute what is meant by a *psychodynamic* view of behavior.

All current behavior is likely to be influenced by our past life experiences. This is true even when we are exposed to new and unique stimuli. It explains why seemingly like individuals exposed to the same current stimulus—a threat, an appeal for help, an opportunity to evade responsibility—will take different and unpredictable paths. It also explains why one individual exposed to seemingly like situations will respond differently and unpredictably. This is a developmental view of behavior.

Human behavior is not random, it is purposive; it is future—as well as past—oriented. We are goal-directed individuals, and once we have passed the struggle for brute survival, our individual goals differ dramatically. We human beings do "work" as well as labor. All animals labor—that is, they engage in the activities to ensure their survival, to obtain food and shelter, and to reproduce. Man and woman alone also work; that is, we create products, artifacts, and works of art to serve our pleasures and our vanities and the peculiar lifestyles that we have evolved beyond caves. We are motivated to acquire the things we create, and we enjoy the mastery of work, the act of creation that we share with our Creator. This is a motivational view of behavior.

Within these behavioral boundaries, people still differ significantly. They differ in their capacity for self-control and self-discipline—their so-called frustration tolerance. They differ in the length of the future they can visualize. For the junkie, the significant future is the moment between injecting the dope and feeling its anticipated pleasure; for the recovering alcoholic, the significant future may be one day at a time. For some accountants, it is the kind of estate planning that (in its attempt to deprive the government of taxes) will disenfranchise the loved children of a rich man by leaving his money through trusts to future generations that he never will know and whom he might despise if he did know them.

In order to understand coercion adequately, one must adopt a dynamic, developmental, and motivational view of behavior. This perspective must also incorporate a notion of unconscious motivation; that is, influences on our action of which we are unaware and that are unacknowledged and often irrational. It is also important to understand the modern psychological view of personhood, which involves the composite of characteristics that make up an individual personality or the self.

The self is where our identity resides. It is the medium through which our actions are guided and our world is perceived. We are often as unaware of its existence as we are of the air around us. This is clear even from dictionary definitions of self: "the total, essential, or particular being of a person," or "the essential qualities distinguishing one person from another," or "one's consciousness of one's own being or identity; the ego."[2]

The self is not a truly autonomous ego, it is an interactive entity defined not just in terms of differences from others but in relationship to them. The answer to the question: "Who are you?" is not satisfied by your stating that you are a woman of forty-three. That much is self-evident; the questioner already knew that. It will usually be answered by such information as: "I am a biologist at Columbia College, working on the problems of immune systems; married to my college sweetheart; I'm a mother of two girls and a boy; I was born in Taiwan but am now a naturalized citizen of the U.S.A.," and on and on and on. The missing ingredient in much discussion of human motivation is exactly the nature of the person, and that requires a complex concept of personhood or self.

What we all tend to share is an unconscious that drives us forward or constrains us, depending on our values and the emotions that support them. This shared unconscious has a direct bearing on public policy and the social uses of coercion. The vain persistence in assuming that all that is necessary to change behavior is to disseminate information (calling it education) is irresponsible leadership. When the life of an individual or the survival of a community depends on those behavioral changes, it is unconscionable to persist in the conceit of a totally rational human being. Yet policymakers continue to act as though drug addiction, dangerous sexual behavior, and crime can be solved by purely cognitive means.

The culture of autonomy stubbornly denies the very psychology that the average person uses in her commonsense approach to her colleagues at work and her children at home. Almost daily we can find evidence of this stubborn self-deception. Consider one more example. Under a headline that reads, "Study Finds that Education Does Not Ease Welfare Rolls," the *New York Times* reports:

> A closely watched experiment in which teenage mothers were show-ered with education and social services had no effect in moving them from welfare into the job market, according to a study made public today. . . . The program, called New Chance, served 1,408 teenagers in 10 states. But after 18 months, those who joined the program were no more likely to be off welfare or in a job than a similar group that received no services. About 80 percent of the mothers from both groups were still collecting welfare, and only 26 percent had worked in the last three months. . . . The program failed to raise actual literacy, with the average woman in both groups still reading below the eighth-grade level. New Chance also did little to raise parenting skills. And it failed to prevent repeat pregnancies, despite counseling and the offers of contraception. About 57 percent of the women in the program got pregnant in the 18 months following

enrollment, compared with 53 percent of the women in the control group.[3]

We cannot take the stuff of knowledge from the hard drive of social
understanding and transfer it to the floppy disk of the individual. Rational,
calculating self-control alone will not sustain the social order essential for
human survival. The social emotions of guilt, shame, and pride are essential
to any society that aspires to be both secure and free. The conditions
necessary to encourage the development of these social emotions, and the
right to exploit them for social and individual good, is thwarted by an
autonomy perspective that would consider all such practices "coercive"
and immoral.

COERCION AS FORCE

Physical force is the prototypical case of coercion, because in most people's
minds it represents the antithesis, or the ultimate abridgement, of autonomy. A whole host of intermediate interventions and social controls that
fall short of physical force—inducements, incentives, enticements, seductions—are less threatening to most people; some that may be more problematic are manipulation and brainwashing. Unfortunately all of the methods
of social control that extend beyond the purely voluntary are tarred with
the broad brush of the vaguely defined adjective *coercive*, often to frighten
the public and to serve political agendas. If we can understand coercion
properly, we will be in a much better position to assess the entire spectrum
for achieving intermediate social control.

Coerce is defined in *The American Heritage Dictionary* as follows: "to
force to act or think in a given manner; to compel by pressure or threat."
This definition is straightforward enough, except that by introducing thinking into the process, it unnecessarily complicates an already confusing
issue. What kind of "force" changes thought? We can force someone to
say that they believe something, but we cannot "force" them to believe it.

Very close to coercion, but for matters of argument best left as a separate
category, is constraint. The second dictionary definition under *coerce* is
essentially a definition of *constraint*: "to dominate, restrain, or control
forcibly." Constraint is a parallel phenomenon to coercion, following all
of the rules of coercion, except that we are not forcing someone *to* do
something they are reluctant to do, but rather constraining them *from*

doing what they wish to do. One reason for separating constraint from coercion is that whereas constraint can well be physical, for all practical purposes coercion cannot be. The generalized misconception of coercion as involving physical force must be laid to rest. Coercion must be perceived as the psychological phenomenon it inevitably is.

In considering the question of coercion there is a natural bias to cling to the physical model. Force is traditionally visualized in physical terms. In this form it is easily definable, clear-cut, and unambiguous. When we turn, however, to concrete examples, it becomes obvious why physical force has minimal significance in any discussion of coercive behavior. Physical force is effective only in inhibiting or preventing action—it can only bind or constrict a person. We can constrain a man from sexual assault, from demonstrating, from pillaging, or indeed from doing almost any activity by locking him up. For the most part in our society, physical constraint is reserved as the privilege of the maintainers of the basic "benevolent" institutions. It is used primarily in hospitals, the family, prisons, and perhaps the schools. It is the parents, the doctor, and the jailer who physically restrain a person, on the supposition that this constraint is in the service of that person or the society.

The psychological dimension of coercion, however, does not involve physical constraint. We can manipulate people (that is, "handle" them) by a whole host of means, thereby bending them to our desires. We can lie to them about our purposes and intentions and deceive them about its effect on them. The simple phrase *informed consent* contains both manipulative and coercive aspects. One must gain the "consent" of the patient to prove that she was not physically or psychologically forced into a procedure. We then insist that this consent be "informed," recognizing that if a patient readily agrees to something about which she understands little or about which she has a false understanding, we have somehow or other abrogated or sidestepped her autonomous decision-making rights.

There is, in addition, a whole spectrum of manipulative and coercive maneuvers that are still short of absolute lying and absolute threat of force. Persuasions, inducements, seductions, and incentives may be either acceptable or unacceptable in their own standing, and although they may be viewed as "coercive," it is important to locate the stops on this continuum that go from "soft" to "hard" coercion. The high salaries of successful lawyers in large firms certainly induce them into working long hours, thereby sacrificing many other things in their lives. Although one might find it odd to say that these lawyers are "coerced" into giving up much time with their families, it is also not fully correct to say that they are acting out of purely free or voluntary choice, either. However we define the gray areas along the spectrum of coercion, the important point is that the location of an action along this spectrum from soft to hard coercion is pertinent to an ethical assessment of that action.

In essence, coercion involves actions that force people to do that which we wish them to do rather than allowing them to do what they wish to do. In other words, in an older language, it involves forcing them to do something "against their will." When we actually transform the will rather than override it, we are in the spectrum of indoctrination to brainwashing. Even when we say that someone is doing what she chooses or wishes to do, the choice may still be weighted with elements that constrain the individual's basic desires or even interests. Human nature does not allow many direct and single moves from desire to deed.

Coercion is forcing someone to act against his will. Like the Ten Commandments, it is oriented toward controlling conduct. Coercion is an instrument of social order and social control. It inhabits the realm of social relationships and institutions. It is as necessary a part of the environment of human behavior as the air we breathe and the light by which we see. To think that coercion could be eliminated from human relationships is a dangerous illusion, one born of theories of autonomy that would like to believe that rational self-control is all that is necessary to maintain social order.

This definition places coercion clearly in the realm of relationships among people, or their institutions. This is where morality itself resides, as William James, that most psychological of philosophers, reminds us:

> Were all other things, gods and men and starry heavens, blotted out from the universe, and were there left but one rock with two loving souls upon it, that rock would have as thoroughly moral a constitution as any possible world which the eternities and immensities could harbor. . . . While they lived there would be real good things and real bad things in the universe; there would be obligations, claims, and expectations; obediences, refusals, and disappointments; compunctions and longings for harmony to come again, and inward

peace of conscience when it was restored; there would, in short, be a moral life.[4]

COERCION BY THREAT

When coercing positive action, physical force can only operate in the smallest range. We can force the movement of a hand or the twisting of a finger, but anything that involves integration and constancy—any purposeful and meaningful behavior—is not coercible on a physical level. We can physically do things to someone; we cannot physically have him do things for us. How do we physically force someone to practice safe sex or avoid driving when drunk?

"Coercion by threat" is that broad domain in which most coercion in the social sense resides. The *threat* of punitive damage is the coercive club—not the *actual* inflicting of damage. Ironically, the threat of physical damage is effective only in its potential form, for once the threat is carried out, it loses its coercive capacity. During the Spanish Inquisition it was the threat of burning, not the actual burning, that brought thousands of "heretics" into the "embrace" of Christianity. An unfired gun pointed at someone's head can force him to act. Once fired, it merely destroys him; it does not induce the desired behavior. Granted, a gun fired at one person can have a coercive effect on another, but here again, firing at one person merely serves to dramatize to the one to be coerced the reality of the threatened danger, and the resolve behind the threat.

This coercive effect of the example of another person's punishment on one's own contemplated behavior is known as *the principle of general deterrence*, one of the five justifying positions for incarceration in the law. Specific deterrence is a second justification for incarceration. (Protection of society, punishment, and rehabilitation are the others.) It is the term reserved for the assumption that the threat of punishment for having transgressed is likely to deter a person from behaving in such a manner again. But the threat of punishment must be perceived as a real threat.

In these situations it is always the potential that dictates behavior; to appreciate the potential, one must be capable of visualizing the future. In their unparalleled capacity for anticipation and visualization, in their ability to learn by experience, in their awareness of the finiteness of life and the fragility of existence, human beings are uniquely equipped to be coerced. Fear is the extension of pain made possible by this capacity to be anticipa-

tory. As such, fear is an efficient symbolic substitute for pain and a fundamental facilitator of coercion. Guilt and shame serve as well, or better, in
individuals who have the capacity to experience those social emotions.
Because fear requires no indoctrination and is a universal experience, it
is the prototype.

Recent tendencies to deny the deterrent effect of threats of punishment
are unscientific and mischievous. "What good will it do to punish him?"
"Punishment never works." "What is really needed is rehabilitation." These
were the shibboleths of the past forty years. They are all wrong. First,
punishing the criminal may do no good for him, but it may do us good;
wrongdoing that goes unpunished demoralizes a society. Second, punishment may not always deter, but it is often the only thing that will prevent
repeat offenses. Psychotherapy in a prison setting is a notorious failure.

To a cerebral animal like ourselves, symbolic events carry great weight.
We are less bound than other animals by a genetically fixed instinctive
patterning. Nor are we limited to fight or flight when we encounter a
threat. We can bargain. We may avoid a blow by submission, compliance,
and obedience. We can sacrifice our freedom of choice to ransom our
security. Returning to the example of the Jew converted at the stake, his
attendance at Mass the Sunday following his "conversion" would be viewed
by most of us as a coerced action, even though he voluntarily woke, bathed,
dressed, and walked to the church.

Fear has a quantitative range, and the point has been consistently made
in law and philosophy that for behavior to be considered coerced, there
must be some correlation between the severity of the threat a person faces
and the severity of the action that the threat actually represents. The
traditional view of psychoanalysis has also distinguished between normal
anxiety, which is proportionate to a threatening situation, and neurotic
anxiety, which is disproportionate. The fallacy of this distinction becomes
apparent when one thinks in more specific terms, for the perceived severity
of a threat often differs from its actual severity.

If a primitive man is threatened by two other men, one of them a big
man with a big stick and the other a small man with a small pistol, we
would expect that having had no experience with pistols, the primitive
man would respond more readily to the man with the stick. In actuality
there is no question of the greater potential danger to him. We who are
knowledgeable know which weapon is the more potent destroyer.

Similarly, if a pistol is held to the head of a woman and she is warned that the trigger will be pulled unless she performs an act, the legitimacy of the coercion exists, whether that pistol is loaded (a real danger) or is unloaded (no danger at all), for it is not the actuality of the danger but the perception of danger which is the crucial issue. A person is threatened by that which she *perceives* to be dangerous, not necessarily by that which is actually dangerous. Often there will be a direct correlation, but there need not be. A woman raped by a man with a toy gun is still a victim of a coercive assault.

To be coerced, therefore, behavior need be commensurate not with the actual threat but with the perceived threat. One sees this particularly in adolescents, whose value systems are so distorted toward social acceptance and peer approval. It does not matter that life will go on without a date for the prom, or after being cut from the basketball team, or after losing a class election. The shame, disgrace, and humiliation of such events are common precipitating factors in teenage suicides. The fear of being viewed as a coward, of being characterized as "chicken," explains the reckless chances that some teenagers take that also result in senseless deaths each year.

To carry this argument one step further, *danger* will be defined by each individual in terms of his knowledge, life experience, and perceptual distortions. The actual threat must be processed through the machinery of the reactive self to produce the perceived threat. To understand coercion, one must understand not only the explicit threat or danger but the way in which it is perceived—the way it is modified by the knowledge, needs, and experience of the threatened individual. Actuality—that is, the measurable external stimulus—is only one factor in determining what we perceive. It is our perception that will determine how we act.

The law recognizes that coercion need not involve physical force, and that even the threatened action need not be physical. In this sense the law has often been ahead of the social sciences. Economic loss, social ostracism, and ridicule are all recognized by law in varying contexts as coercive forces.[5]

In a social animal approval and acceptance are almost always perceived as necessary for its very survival. Certain values are perceived as more essential to survival than "living" itself. These values vary according to the culture. During the final stages of World War II, *kamikaze* attacks became an effective weapon for the Japanese. The ritual suicide of the Japanese pilot was not seen as destroying him. Rather, the true death would have been to dishonor the Japanese war effort and the emperor by refusing to fly to his death. It would have been inconceivable for the United States to institutionalize such an action.

Certain symbols, which have a validity and meaning only within the life experience and sensibility of a specific individual, will carry for him the weight and force of a life-endangering experience. Most of the terrors that plague people in daily existence, psychiatrists know, involve these symbolic equivalents of death rather than the actuality. Ironically, such people handle the actuality of death itself, for the most part, by denying its very existence. To understand coercion, one must understand that which threatens the human being. We must consider all the sources of fear, guilt, and shame.

COERCION AS INDOCTRINATION

Thus far we have been dealing with the kinds of force, threats, and emotions that operate in the conscious awareness of the person being coerced. What about manipulating an individual by "speaking" directly to the unconscious? Such manipulation introduces the possibility of an alternative kind of coercion involving covert or simply unarticulated mechanisms. This coercion would not simply involve forcing a person to do that which you want (as distinguished from what he wants) but rather forcing him, through the manipulation of his emotions, to *will* what you want him to will. When you exploit the anxieties of a person rather than his reason—and this may be done either with or without his awareness—you are coercing his behavior, often without either the recognition or admission of coercion on either side.

The power to coerce is the power to control a person's tacit frame of reference. No better example of an implicit coercive power exists than the power of medicine to force behavior to conform to a standard merely by defining it as either sick or healthy. Oliver Wendell Holmes, himself a physician, recognized this principle in the days when medicine was all promise and no performance:

There is nothing people will not do, there is nothing they have not done, to recover their health and save their lives. They have submitted to be half drowned in water, half cooked with gases, to be buried up to their chins in earth, to be seared with hot irons like slaves, to be crimped with knives, like codfish, to have needles thrust into their flesh, and bonfires kindled on their skin, to swallow all sorts of abominations, and to pay for all this, as if to be singed and scaled were a costly privilege, as if blisters were a blessing and leeches were a luxury.[6]

Psychoanalysis and psychiatry, as the parts of medicine that deal with conduct, have had an undue, highly leveraged influence on modern moral behavior. They have been unusually effective in influencing behavior (particularly in the United States) through their power to label behavior as either "normal" and therefore desirable and acceptable, or "abnormal" and thus undesirable and unapproved. They introduced a new way of ordering and integrating individual and group behavior, and in the process certain value judgments became seriously changed.

A new therapeutic ethic was introduced without being so defined. Things that were formerly seen as perverse—in the sexual area, for example—now became normal. The unnatural became natural. Psychoanalysis liberated whole areas of behavior from the domain of religion and morality and redefined them in medical terms. A piece of behavior, like a wart, could now be seen as sick or healthy. The implications of this shift were not immediately apparent.

Consider the ubiquitous self-entertainment called masturbation. Prior to the nineteenth century masturbation (onanism) was considered a sin. When our culture turned away from the moral authority of the church, the word *sin* was practically dropped from the average person's vocabulary. Masturbation was then deemed vaguely immoral. When Freud suggested that all people masturbate, particularly in childhood, such masturbation became accepted as normal; only the persistence of masturbation into adult life was labeled as neurotic or sexually immature—and then only if it was narcissistically preferred to sexual intercourse. Starting in the 1970s, when radical feminists perceived heterosexual sex as a form of female enslavement, they defined masturbation as a force for liberation and a political act; a *failure* to masturbate was now viewed as a neurotic inhibition. Thus our attitudes about masturbation by an adult "progressed" (if that is the proper term) from sinful to immoral to immature to liberated—that is, superhealthy!

Some may see this change as purely semantic, and therefore insignificant: we changed only the name of the game, and health simply became the new morality. But this view is a dangerous underestimation; in changing the name, we changed much more. We changed the venue, we changed the frame of reference, and we also changed the rules of the game, the locus of authority, and the relationship between the expert and the lay person.

The unparalleled power that we place in the hands of doctors stems directly from that existential fear of death that we all share. The preserver of life has often been exempted from normal rules of behavior in the service of his profession. This exemption holds whether he is a priest or physician, and there have been times when both have literally gotten away with murder. Changing of the frame of reference from a religious to a medical one has had a profound impact on controlling individual action.

Today, if a priest informs us that divorce, or contraception, or eating meat on Friday is sinful and prohibited, we are more likely to change our religion than change our behavior. A higher percentage of Catholic women have abortions in the United States than do non-Catholic women. However, there are certain areas where our outlook approaches unanimity. Health is the one polarity that most approximates the absolute on the scale of desirability. No person aspires to sickness (at least no "healthy" person), for sickness is the prelude to death. We are frightened of sickness. That is why we may listen to our lawyer's "counsel," but we tend to follow our doctor's "orders." By defining specific conduct as either healthy or sick, psychiatrists have had a profound effect in directing individuals' behavior—although with an unbelievable conceit they have claimed a neutral stand in the field of morals.

Victorian morality, which was supported by traditional theology and unchallenged by any countervailing psychology, presumed that sexual pleasure was "unnatural" for women of character. In those days of "wifely duties" a woman often saw her own frigidity as a matter of pride, a symbol of refinement, a statement of virtue, as did others. To this day women are striving to free themselves from this erroneous stereotype. Now that it is deemed healthy for women to enjoy sexuality, a psychoanalyst is often in the peculiar position of indicating to a woman that she has the privilege of refusing sexual advances—that it is not "sick" to not always be sexually receptive. This is but one example of how psychiatry and psychoanalysis have become major factors in defining acceptable or permissible behavior without accepting the responsibility of examining the social implications of such behavior.

Another example is our still-unresolved attitude toward homosexuality, which has traditionally been condemned in most religions. Freud attempted to lift the moral bias against homosexuality by referring to it as simply a sexual deviation (literally a *de via*, "another path") or a perversion (from *pervere*, "to turn away") from the norm. Needless to say, this redefinition offered little comfort to homosexuals. *Pervert* and *deviant* quickly took on pejorative meanings that, if anything, added greater burdens to the homosexual life. Now traditional psychoanalysis has taken a different stance on homosexuality, labeling it as simply an alternative in sexual "object choice." This is another oversimplification. Homosexuality represents a different set of values, a different priority of motives, and a different culture from heterosexuality, as male and female homosexuality are also different (often antithetically) from each other.

These examples all point in the same direction. When a traditional moral or religious authority defines a specific behavior as immoral, people today—particularly in a heterogeneous society where such authorities conflict—often feel perfectly free to accept or reject that authority. If, however, a medical authority defines the same behavior as "healthy," the individual will *wish* to engage in it; we all want to be healthy. If a medical authority labels something "unhealthy," it is avoided. In both cases, people willingly conform their behavior to the definitions of the medical authority. They embrace sexual freedom; try to avoid high-fat diets; exercise to the point of tedium; vent their spleen rather than repressing their rage; accept the "feminine" or "masculine" side of their personality, as the case may be.

The use of coercion to transform a person's will and to alter his frame of reference is also documented in the practices of psychiatry and psychotherapy. Psychiatry, a branch of medicine, is trapped between its goals, which are defined by medicine, and its methodology, which clings stubbornly to a model of education. Psychotherapy has been defined by many as a form of reeducation. After all, although it is behavior that psychiatrists are dealing with, their methods are often simply talking to a patient. But even when they only talk to a patient, more is going on through the transference than the patient, and often the doctor, realizes. Any psychiatrist who tries to convince a patient to give up his fear of subways or elevators via logical arguments about the safety of both methods of transport is likely to be countered by the angry retort: "You don't have to tell me it's crazy to be so afraid. If I didn't know that already, what the hell would I be doing in a psychiatrist's office!"

Whatever psychiatrists claim to do, their practice certainly involves emotional reconditioning, a form of manipulation that actually bypasses cognitive processes. When the psychiatrist hears of a piece of behavior of which he disapproves, he labels it as "sick," "neurotic," "maladaptive," or "dysfunctional." Similarly, he labels desired behavior as "healthy" or "adaptive." In this way, both patient and analyst can operate under the conceit that no pressure is exerted on the patient to make his behavior conform to the doctor's demands. This preserves the untenable notion of a value-free medicine.

Instead, the doctor should unapologetically recognize and announce that she has a set of values that she is promoting, the values implicit in the definition of health. A doctor does not serve her patient's desires— what if he wished to be a happy drug addict, or schizophrenic? Rather, she serves a set of values that she and her culture and the majority of her patients share. These values are defined as "health," and she is a minister in the service of that value system.

Through the power of transference (a patient's trust and feeling for the doctor; the desire to please her), the patient is driven toward healthy, nondestructive behavior: toward work over indolence, activity over passivity, involvement over isolation, pleasure over pain. What is wrong with this effort? Because it is directed—as it usually is—toward increasing the power and freedom of the patient, should we even care that a form of unconscious manipulation is occurring—particularly because both doctor and patient may be deceived into thinking otherwise?

It is not possible here to analyze the entire methodology of psychotherapy, but we must recognize that it is a less intellectual procedure than most would suspect. It involves emotional manipulations and coercive forces. And it is a worthy enterprise. By any definition, a psychotherapist enhances the ultimate capacity of a patient to exercise autonomy, even though the process itself clearly bypasses the patient's autonomy in ways that he—or even his therapist—may not fully realize.

This is not to say that speaking to the unconscious is either better or worse than other forms of coercion. One cannot make a judgment on the morality of any form of coercion without knowing the nature of the behavior it produces, or the identity and the purposes of the individual contributing to the behavior. What the psychoanalyst does is closely related to what the good parent does. Often the therapist is, indeed, undoing the maladaptive lessons of childhood.

In rearing children our goal is to have a child who *chooses* to do good, rather than one who does the right thing only out of fear of punishment. We want a child to share his toys out of his own sense of generosity, not out of his fear of our disapproval. But parents can instill generosity in children only by making negative responses to their selfishness and positive responses to their sharing. The mechanisms of conscience that generate good behavior are for the most part products of direct speaking to the unconscious, on a level that, were it conscious, would be called coercive.

We do not condemn this method of indoctrination—little good it would do us—because it is in the service of the good, and because the agents are parents and their children. Once again, when we judge the moral basis of coercion, we find no absolute guidelines based on methodology.

In this example, it is the relationship of the coerced individual to the coercer that defines the moral good. In the parent-child relationship direct appeals to the unconscious are the methods of choice. Parents try to create a child who does good, without threatening him or explicitly instructing him to do good.

COERCION AS BRAINWASHING

It is revealing to examine the differences in our attitudes toward the moral indoctrination of the young and the psychoanalytic "reeducation" of the neurotic, on the one hand, and toward the notion of "brainwashing," on the other. In psychotherapy such unconscious manipulation is acceptable to some and not to others. When psychological manipulation is done beneficently—for the patient's good—and when patient and therapist share the definition of it as good, it is unlikely even to be defined as coercion. But when the same type of unconscious manipulation is a calculated policy of the powerful state against the individual citizen, an almost universal condemnation can be expected. When it occurs in a prisoner of war camp or even in a "revolutionary college," we will label the same manipulations as brainwashing.

Sometimes it is difficult to say whether coercion is actively maintained or passively perpetuated. What one group sees as an accidental development, another may view as conspiracy. Think of the prototypes and stereotypes of the white majority and their influence on African American self-images and self-esteem. In a traditional sense, no one "forced" African Americans to straighten their hair. No one forced them to use skin lighteners or to be ashamed of "black" features. But in a society in which white was right and only white was beautiful—a society that in addition was highly competitive, rewarding winners lavishly and punishing losers severely—African Americans were forced to want to be white, an impossible task leading to self-denial, self-humiliation, and self-abasement.

To belong to a group, to be acceptable, to be lovable, is psychologically equated with being worthy, safe, and secure. This form of coercion was of course helped along by a white society that could permit the "whitest" of African Americans to enjoy privileges, economic and otherwise, that were denied the "blacker" ones.

The "black is beautiful" movement rightly recognized the coercive effect of the majority prototype. It was a profound insight to recognize that the majority prototype was a club that had been used to beat the African Americans into submission. Its coercive impact, incidentally, is just as great, whether it was designed to produce the effect or whether the effect was an accidental historic and developmental spin-off. Even if this prototype was not a part of a conspiracy to subjugate the minority, it was still coercive. But is it brainwashing or indoctrination? And if we invent prototypes that are designed to *counter* racial stereotypes, but operate in the same way, and if we consciously disseminate this information, is that indoctrination, reeducation, or brainwashing? The state can, of course, rectify past injustice by using legal sanctions against racism (coercion in the service of the good). Is one form of coercion necessarily superior to the other? Does employing the latter preclude our also employing the former?

In some cases brainwashing has been conscious, overt, and calculated, with the presence of the coercer obvious, as practiced by the Chinese in the Korean war. Even if it could be demonstrated that the brainwashers injected nothing into their subjects, that they used no physical torture, the practice would still be universally condemned. One suspects that it is precisely when no physical agents are used that brainwashing is most threatening. The very impalpability of the agents enhances our sense of vulnerability; the unknowable anxiety is always the greatest dread. Posthypnotic suggestion mystifies and frightens most people, particularly in the exaggerated claims of fiction, as in the acclaimed novel and movie *The Manchurian Candidate*.[7]

Although disgust at and rejection of brainwashing is general in this country, it should be remembered that the term is specifically American and always refers to something that other people do. The Chinese term for the same form of coercion was much less malignant: they called it "ideological thought reform," and already, willy-nilly, it seemed less threatening. This coercion, as the Chinese now employ it, is not limited to prisoners of war or to a prison setting. It has been applied to questionable students, wayward political figures, and stubborn teachers. When it was applied to these groups, it was done in a "revolutionary college," which brings it back to the respectable area of education. In his writings on the subject, Mao Zedong used a medical analogy to explain the goals of thought reform:

> Our object in exposing errors and criticizing shortcomings is like that of a doctor in curing a disease. The entire purpose is to save the person, not to cure him to death. If a man has an appendicitis the doctor performs an operation and the man is saved. If a person who commits an error, no matter how great, does not bring his disease to an incurable stage by concealing it and persisting in his error, in addition, if he is genuinely and honestly willing to be cured, willing to make corrections, we will welcome him so that his disease may be cured and he can become a good comrade. . . . We . . . must have an attitude of saving men by curing their diseases. This is the correct and effective method.[8]

The Chinese see the revolutionary college as an educative institution, an institution for the good. But this type of coercion is not limited to the Chinese and need not be performed in such a blatant way.

The purpose of all propaganda, and indoctrination, is not to force a man to *do* that which others will, but rather, through manipulation of his emotions, to force him to *will* that which others will. Such indoctrination is as common in the West as it is in Asia. Consider psychoanalysis once again. It is morally supported by the fact that the patient himself already subscribes to the conviction that his symptoms need changing; they are already anathema to him—"ego-alien," the psychoanalyst would label them. But some of the sickest patients—manic-depressives or paranoids, for example—do not view themselves or their symptoms as "sick." The psychoanalyst's first step is to try to alienate such a patient from his symptoms—to convince him that the voices are not real, that the plot against him is imaginary.

Or consider the field of advertising, which is based on a growing science of propaganda and an established methodology of promotion and salesmanship. Today little soap is sold on the basis of its cleansing power, now that it has been proven that the more effective sales pitch is to convince the consumer that he will "offend" if he does not use the safeguarding brand. Scientific salesmanship has long recognized the superiority of coercive fear over logic as a means of persuasion. Moreover, it has learned that fear is not as difficult to effect as one might presume. "Motivational research experts" can be hired, like accountants, to assist in the task, and increasing amounts of advertising budgets are going into such marketing research.

Advertising can be exploited equally to sell a president as to sell a pill.[9] In the area of personalities of candidates, salesmanship is of limited effectiveness. The intimacy of television allows the candidate's real personality to seep through any packaging. But in terms of programs and plans (health care packages, AIDS policies, the genome project) about which voters are unknowledgeable and unsure, salesmanship can be potent and decisive. Coercion is usually quicker and surer than education, and if coercion is to be used in national politics, generating fear is more efficient than applying physical force in mobilizing masses of people.

The field of advertising is currently the prime arena of speaking directly to the unconscious. Nowhere is this form of coercion more apparent than in the cigarette industry's Joe Camel and Marlboro Man advertising campaigns. Some ads are aimed directly at the insecurities and aspirations of adolescent boys. Others are aimed specifically at the insecurities and aspirations of teenage girls. And they work. Studies have clearly indicated that teenagers gravitate to these brands in disproportionate numbers. Making appeal to the emotions and directly addressing the unconscious work.

How odd that we allow manipulation to be used to addict large segments of our population to cigarettes, but we resort to ineffectual "education" in attempting to remove addiction—an immeasurably more difficult task.

In any society, manipulating through the unconscious represents both a threat and an opportunity. It is a particular threat to a free society because it can operate without the knowledge of the person being manipulated— even with the appearance of his consent. As such, manipulation through the unconscious is a form of coercion that is free to operate under the old definitions, or illusions, of autonomy. But it is also the device of choice in the parental guidance of children. By appealing to pride, shame, and guilt, a parent not only shapes a child's specific behavior at the moment but helps to develop the internal constraints on antisocial behavior that lie at the core of conscience. Here the sphere of operation and the identity and relationship of the agents become crucial in defining the morality of the procedure.

COERCION AND THE COMMON GOOD

The parent-child relation is a special case that allows for intrusion on personal autonomy at its extreme. But surely such bypassing of rationality would be permissible in adults to some extent as well. We do it anyhow. By establishing our cultural heroes, we set models for emulation. Few people actively pattern after these models by conscious decision. It "happens." We just seem to become something like them. Changing the nature of our heroes, and how they are defined, could be one constructive approach to solving some of our social problems. There is no reason that antismoking campaigns should not use the proven methodology of cigarette (and other) advertising, even though it manipulates people emotionally and hardly aims to make them more autonomous. We need not be even-handed in our use of these techniques in the service of public health and the common good. We might well ban manipulative advertising for cigarettes but approve it for antismoking campaigns.

Justice and the good demand that we have a better understanding of the limits of autonomy. These concepts are sufficiently complex to demand more elements in their construction than simply autonomy. We must reexamine our prejudices. We must change certain behaviors for the benefit of a good society, a society that aspires to nurture all its citizens to their fullest potential for a good life. And we must use the full range of encouragements and restraints that an understanding of motivation has made available.

Politics, human nature, moral philosophy, and psychology are inextricably linked when we enter the world of social change. Underlying all political discussions is a set of psychological assumptions that are generally unarticulated or, worse, unacknowledged. Americans routinely criticize the state of our governmental and corporate institutions. We abhor the lack of politesse in our public behavior. We despair at the lawlessness in our streets. We observe with a sense of helplessness the rise in drug addiction and the spread of AIDS. We decry the indolence of youth, the greed of politicians, the selfishness of the affluent, and the corruptibility of the power brokers. When we make these objections, we are making a political statement. We are tacitly enunciating a set of values that define the way we think things ought to be. We are, if only negatively, defining the good society. We are also making basic assumptions about human motivation, and too often these assumptions are incorrect. The culture of autonomy has ignored that which we know, or should know, about human psychology, in order to preserve a particular political view of human behavior as self-chosen and rational.

Appeals to emotion—even when they are admitted to be more effective—are persistently and stubbornly viewed as morally inferior to appeals to reason. Surely, many Americans believe, appealing to a person's honor, his unselfishness, and his hidden sense of duty is a way of bringing his better self forward. Why shouldn't we make people feel ashamed of littering? Guilty about their vulgarity and rudeness? Humiliated to be seen urinating in public spaces? And if an appeal to the primitive emotion of fear is the only effective way to summon a person's better self, what's wrong with that? Why shouldn't we make a man as afraid to assault his wife as he is to assault a policeman? More important, when we know rationality alone cannot work, there is something duplicitous and self-deceiving in our insistence on utilizing it exclusively.

"Just say no," the rationalist advises. To drugs, sex, and alcohol? Just say no—to greed, police graft, and political corruption? Whom are we kidding? "No parking" signs are less effective than the presence of a policeman with a summons book. In some societies the summons is unnecessary. In Switzerland a doorman will chastise publicly a cab driver who carelessly drops a cigarette butt on the public sidewalk, and the shame will be visible on the driver's face. Unfortunately, in this aspect, New York is not Zurich; nor is London, Paris, Madrid, or Tel Aviv.

Even if appeals to reason were morally "superior," what might we do about the kinds of behavior that seem immune to reason: behavior driven by greed, fear, rage, envy, selfishness, and paranoia? What can possibly be immoral about helping a person overcome those drives that damage himself, as well as people around him, by enlisting emotions such as guilt and shame? For that matter, what is wrong with reinforcing his better self by raising a countervalent fear through threat of disapproval or punishment?

Coercive and manipulative attempts to change behavior are not unjust or wrong per se. But why do we so often assume that they are? And how can we differentiate those instances of coercion and social control that are ethically justified from those that are not? It is to the ethical assessment of coercion that we now turn.

9

In Defense of Social Control:
The Ethics of Coercion

Social order is by no means a mere hive or herd order.
It seems to be a *fabric*, rather than a *growth*. But, in any
case, it is important to know what human nature can
furnish in the cause of social harmony. The gulf between
private ends and public ends, between the aims of the
individual and his fellows, is bridged from both sides, and
we must know what abutments and spans are provided by
the individual himself, if we are to measure the extent
of the moral engineering that must be undertaken by
society.

—EDWARD ALSWORTH ROSS, *Social Control*

FIN-DE-SIÈCLE AMERICA WAS a curiously introspective and nervous society,
and the first few years of the new century do not seem to have changed
that. We have "won" the cold war, and our political and economic institutions are imitated and admired around the world. And yet we worry end-
lessly about whether the future will be better or worse than the past.
Terrorism and economic recession have not helped. In many ways the
world seems a more dangerous and incomprehensible place than ever. The
pax Americana promises to be studded by local and regional conflicts into
which we will be drawn.

Growing numbers of people believe the future will be worse, regardless
of social class or income scale, except perhaps at its very top-most rungs.
People in poverty or on its margins have been hard hit since 1980; they
believe things are getting worse because they are.[1] Middle-class Americans,
whose economic standard of living has been pretty much stagnant since
the 1970s, feel exhausted by the race to stay in place; they doubt that the

social promises of private pensions, Social Security, and Medicare will be there for them in their old age, and they doubt that their children will do better than they have done.

These fears may sometimes be exaggerated, but they are certainly not unreasonable. Certain undeniable facts of American life—racism, poverty, crime, drug abuse, violence, broken families, neglected children, poor public education—are universally decried. But on and on they go, year after year, apparently beyond our collective ability or will to change. Why? Is it because the problems are simply too large and complex? Or is it because America has become such a diverse society that it is impossible to achieve any effective consensus on what our public goals should be?

Such explanations do not get to the heart of the problem, in our view. America has not lost its capacity to tell the difference between right and wrong. The problem is not one of moral awareness but one of social and political will. Our society currently knows what is right but cannot bring itself to do it. "Things fall apart, the center cannot hold," wrote poet William Butler Yeats in an Ireland torn by civil war.[2] The relevant question for us is less drastic but no less consequential. It is not whether the American center will hold but whether it can act. Can we take steps to shape and control behavior in society to turn the tide on today's destructive trends? If so, how would we publicly and ethically justify doing it?

Americans have for too long neglected and disparaged the mechanisms of social control. We have all but lost the moral vocabulary, the conceptual framework, by which coercive measures can be justified. By "mechanisms of social control," we mean both formal mechanisms, like the law and the police, and the informal mechanisms of culture and society, such as mores, social pressures, and character-forming socialization processes. Can we rely upon these institutions of social control as they now stand? Do they need repair, and if so which ones, and how do we repair them? If we strengthen social controls, will we endanger our freedom? How can coercion be used in a proper, legitimate, morally justified way?

As we contemplate these and similar questions, few among us today are likely to be as sanguine as Archibald MacLeish (quoted in chapter 2) in believing that our country can do virtually anything it sets its mind to. Some do continue to envision what MacLeish called the "unimagined America," the better America that is yet to be. Others are preoccupied with what might be called the "unimaginable America," the frightening image of breakdown, declining standards of living, polarization, and violence. It is wise to keep both the unimagined and the unimaginable in mind. People are beginning to question seriously whether our institutions of social control are adequate and whether the moral, legal, and political constraints against social control and coercion are too sweeping and too stringent.

Our thesis can be stated in the following terms: The culture of autonomy does not permit and cannot adequately justify the means of social control that are necessary to sustain social order and indeed to sustain individual autonomy itself. Autonomy does not give us the conceptual tools we need to think intelligently and decide appropriately about social policies and practices that have a controlling or coercive effect on individual behavior. We must reach beyond the philosophical and psychological framework of autonomy to understand properly the ethics of social control and the proper uses of coercion in a liberal society.

To say that we must reach beyond the culture of autonomy in order to assess social control and coercion as moral issues is not to say that the liberal philosophical tradition can be jettisoned or swept aside. But the way in which autonomy understands social control and coercion, and the limited way it is prepared ethically to justify them, are often insufficient. Here a proposition we put forward earlier bears repeating: There can be no free society without individual autonomy, and there can be no sustainable society that rests on autonomy alone.

APPROACHING COERCION FROM AN ETHICAL POINT OF VIEW

Having discussed the psychological bases of coercion and the interpersonal shaping of behavior in preceding chapters, our task now is to examine the ethical justification of social control and—what amounts to the same thing—the ethical limits of individual autonomy. The philosophical literature on coercion is large and approaches vary.[3] We will not discuss these debates in detail, but will focus on five factors crucial to the ethical assessment of acts of coercion:

1. *agency*—who or what is exercising control over the individual's behavior;

2. *intent*—to what purpose control is being exercised;

3. *consequence*—the outcome or effect of the exercise of control or coercion;

4. *means*—the type of coercion that is being used, the social or psychological means through which it operates, and whether it is proportionate to the goal being sought;

5. *context*—the setting or circumstances in which coercion takes place.

A police officer threatening a civil rights demonstrator with a raised nightstick is not the same as a night rider burning a cross on the front lawn of the new African American family on the block, or a skinhead painting a swastika on the door of a Jewish home. And neither of these acts of coercion is the same as an IRS audit, a seatbelt or motorcycle helmet law, a town curfew ordinance or truancy law, an office dress code, or a community program in which parents sign a pledge to ban alcoholic beverages at teenage parties in their homes. In short, different spheres of society present different circumstances and ethical standards relevant to trade-offs between autonomy and coercion and social control.

This variegation seems to us quite proper and reasonable. It suggests neither ethical relativism nor an outlook of "situation ethics." Rather, it follows from the fact that different spheres and settings in society, such as the state, the institutions of civil society (like churches, neighborhood groups, voluntary organizations), and the family all have their own traditions, codes of behavior, and ethical expectations. The culture of autonomy, as we have seen, has grown out of the transformation of political liberalism into social liberalism and an expansion of the paradigm governing the relationship between the individual and the state to cover all relationships and areas of social life. The result has been a growing tendency to use "coercion" as a simple synonym for "the abuse of power" and to judge instances of coercion in all social spheres as though they were the same as coercion by the state.

These bad habits of civic and moral discourse have made people inattentive to precisely those factors of agency, intent, consequence, means, and context that an ethical analysis of coercion should highlight. Once these factors are clarified, it is possible to examine particular institutional or public policies designed to control individual behavior in coercive ways. In the final section of this chapter and in chapter 10 we discuss several such cases and indicate how this framework of ethical analysis can be applied to issues such as drug use by pregnant women, parental responsibility for adolescent criminal behavior, and the medical treatment and legal responsibility of the mentally ill.

In chapter 13 we shall explore how the culture of autonomy, and the liberal tradition from which it comes, allows for and even justifies social control and coercion under certain circumstances. Autonomy is not opposed to obedience, as long as it is based on an autonomous decision to obey. Autonomy is not opposed to rules, as long as they are restraints and limits that the individual imposes on himself for good reasons. In particular, autonomy allows for coercion and social control when the freedom of one individual must be limited so that the freedom of other individuals can be promoted.

Theorists of autonomy generally permit such restraints when the exercise of one person's freedom will do harm to others. In other cases, autonomy in one sense may be sacrificed in order to protect autonomy in a different sense. For example, autonomy in the sense of independence may conflict with autonomy as negative liberty or freedom from danger or indignity. This conflict of autonomy with itself, so to speak, may arise among two or more people, or within the life of a single individual. In a nursing home, for example, the independence of one resident to watch television late at night may conflict with the privacy and the negative liberty of other residents. In another case, the parent of a seriously disabled person may resist her son's desire to move to a group home because she believes that he would be taken advantage of by the proprietors there. Generally speaking, when a conflict arises within the values most esteemed by the concept of autonomy, it is negative liberty that prevails. When coercion and social control are ethically justified in the culture of autonomy, it is only to prevent harm and to protect the negative liberty or negative rights of one person against others.

The prevention of harm and the protection of negative liberty are not sufficient in and of themselves, however, to establish the moral limits of autonomy. We must be able to justify social control over individual behavior on the basis of values other than preventing harm. Some behaviors are wrong and should be socially controlled because they are wrong, not because they are harmful. And sometimes limits on autonomy are necessary not so much for negative reasons—because they prevent harm or protect the right to be left alone—as for positive reasons: social control can promote the good of the individual and can help sustain relationships of community and commitment with others. Beyond autonomy, the human good involves relationships of interdependence, reciprocity, mutual aid, and serving a value or goal greater than oneself.

Moral reasoning of this kind transcends the language of autonomy and the conceptual framework of liberalism. In fact, as Americans consider social policy, they often realize that it does, but the language of autonomy is so familiar that they try to use prevention of harm to others as the rationale for rules or policies that limit individual freedom of choice. This bad habit of civic discourse frequently leads to ethically distorted arguments and sometimes to dishonest or at least disingenuous ones. At other times, it leaves us only a stuttering and wooden tongue with which to express the moral importance of relationships and commitments in our lives. For a being whose nature is to be social, the language of autonomy, rights, and negative liberty does not even begin to describe our moral possibilities and our moral responsibilities.

Social Order, Social Control, and Coercion

It is impossible to imagine a truly human—let alone humane—society without social order. Attempts to do so, such as thought experiments in social theory or anthropological descriptions of cultures at the extreme point of breakdown, only prove the rule. Consider the war of all against all in Hobbes's state of nature—where one must live in constant fear and insecurity.[4] Or the arbitrary, capricious, maddening world ruled by the Queen of Hearts in Lewis Carroll's Wonderland.[5] Or the miserable life of starvation, selfishness, and mutual indifference among the Ik tribe of northern Uganda, as described by anthropologist Colin Turnbull.[6] All of these societies (two imaginary, one real) lack social order. Each is a place where the most distinctively human aspects of life cannot survive. These aspects are meaning, coherence, predictability, stability, and continuity; social order makes them possible. Order in society, no less than in nature, gives us confidence in the connection between cause and effect, between what is fitting here and now and what is not. Without these things we are lost.

If no society can be human without order, it is possible nonetheless that an orderly society can exist without either social control or coercion. Social order is not the same as social control; the coercive mechanisms of social control, as we use the term here, are but one means among several to achieve or sustain social order. But they are essential and indispensable means, as we shall see.

Social order without social control is possible, at least in theory, because each individual might spontaneously coordinate his behavior with that of all others to form a pattern—what the early economists called a "natural harmony of interests."[7] Social control involves some force—whether "external" and institutional, or "internal" and psychological—operating on the behavior of individuals, giving that behavior direction and coordination that the individuals being influenced may or may not be aware of and may or may not prefer. The behavior of many individuals can spontaneously fall into some kind of coordinated pattern without social control, as when people coming into an auditorium without ushers fill the seats from the center toward the rear of the hall first; only when the back half of the auditorium is full do they move toward the front.

Social order exists without social control in the instinctually determined behavior of animals and humans as well. Each spider of a certain species will spin an intricate and unique web pattern according to the genetic programming of its kind, without any orders from other spiders, without any instruction, and without any published web-spinning guide. Salmon will swim upstream to spawn, without any institution or mechanism of social control, and yet to the outside observer their behavior is of great order, coherence, and continuity. Almost all neurologically normal human infants will smile at twelve to fifteen weeks of age (about when the charming novelty of having a newborn is wearing thin for the mother), regardless of culture and almost regardless of prior adult reactions or stimulation.

One interesting example of social order without social control occurs when individuals consciously and rationally direct their behavior to achieve cooperation and coordination. They are acting intentionally, so the pattern that results is neither spontaneous nor instinctual. In contrast to the way a crowd fills an auditorium, consider the behavior of drivers at a highway toll plaza, or shoppers at a supermarket checkout area. In such cases of queuing, it is not efficient for some lines to be long and others short; to keep the toll-takers busy and to move people through the gates in the shortest period of time, the lines should be as equal as possible.

Now, this coordination problem could be solved by means of social control. There could be police directing traffic into various lanes some distance ahead of the toll plaza. Or some electronic monitoring device could direct each person to a particular lane or the shortest line. (Such a system is used at some railroad-station ticket windows.) But the commonest way to handle this coordination problem is not by means of directive command or coercive social control but by means of voluntary selection based upon self-interest. In most highway toll plazas or supermarkets each driver or shopper scans the situation ahead and maneuvers into the shortest line. Everyone wants to move through as quickly as possible, and when each person picks the shortest line, all the lines tend to remain roughly equal.

This is an everyday example of order and coordination based on voluntary autonomous choice. It is what is generically called a "market mechanism." Proponents of autonomy, especially libertarians, would like to generalize this method of social coordination throughout social life. However, there is no reason to think that this is possible; behavior guided by voluntary preferences of individuals will not necessarily realize even the value of efficiency—as it seems to in the case of queuing behavior—let alone other values, such as justice, mutual aid, community, and beneficence.

Virtually all societies normally sustain social order by means of social control. Social control always involves coercion, although it does not always require physical force. Coercion, it may be recalled, is a social phenomenon beyond physical force. It requires the capacity to anticipate the result of a threatened action on one's life. Lower animals cannot be threatened—they can only be forced or constrained. Higher animals, to the degree that they have instincts of self-preservation and the emotion of fear, can be coerced. Once a pecking order has been established, it is obeyed, but no creature comes close to humans in the extent, ubiquity, and complexity of the coercion we employ on one another.

Coercion changes behavior by working on the emotions of an individual, operating through his rational and executive self. Appeals to the social emotions of guilt, shame, and pride are the most complex and the most interesting mechanisms of coercion as a means of social control. We believe that it is easier to justify social coercion ethically, and easier to reconcile it with autonomy, when it is based on the social as opposed to the primitive emotions. Fear and anger are costly and unnecessarily oppressive instruments of social control; they must be used sparingly and judiciously in an open society.

Herein lies the tragic irony of the culture of autonomy. By failing to appreciate the moral and psychological importance of the social emotions of guilt, shame, pride, and conscience, and by undermining the coercive institutions that develop and sustain them, the culture of autonomy is paving the way for more repressive and authoritarian forms of social control in the long run. Social order is too important to human beings to do without; nature does not provide it for us by instinct, and it cannot emerge in a purely voluntary or spontaneous way, like the invisible hand of the market. Therefore, social order must be maintained on the basis of some degree of social control and coercion. The only real question is what kind of coercion it will be and on what psychological foundations it will rest.

The social emotions are psychologically powerful enough to actually change and direct individual behavior, yet by operating *within and through* the self rather than *on* the self, they respect autonomy, at least to a degree. By allowing individuals to act on their own, the social emotions maintain the moral responsibility and integrity of the individual.

Consider two literary examples. Left to himself, the hero of Stephen Crane's *The Red Badge of Courage* would not fight, but shame, honor, and pride prove to be powerfully motivating and coercive elements in his existential struggle.[8] An analogous example that leads to a more complicated resolution is found in Mark Twain's *Adventures of Huckleberry Finn.*[9] Huck Finn on his own is about as uncorrupted and unbigoted a character as any to be found in literature. But he struggles against feelings growing out of the racist cultural code of his society that he has internalized. When he helps Jim, the runaway slave, escape down the river, he is overwhelmed with guilt. After all, he has broken the rules respected by the "civilized" people in his community. Guilt and conventional morality nearly coerce Huck into turning Jim over to the white authorities. But in the end his natural sympathy and affection for Jim prevail. His wise and compassionate heart identifies with Jim. He perceives him as a human being like himself, defying the social conventions that would use Jim's surface identity as an excuse to define him as an inferior being.

With wonderful irony, Twain has Huck's struggle with his conscience conclude in a kind of resigned self-condemnation. Because he cannot bring himself to do the obviously "right" thing and turn Jim in, Huck finally decides that he is a hopelessly incorrigible person, unfit for membership in the society of civilized folk.

In Huck's case, coercion operating through the social emotions is present on two levels. At one level, Huck rejects the pressure of a guilty conscience springing from his upbringing in a racist society. But Huck Finn overcomes the code of his society not by some rational exercise of pure autonomy but by the influence of another moral order—a natural sense of rightness and goodness deep within him. Read in this way, *Adventures of Huckleberry Finn* is one of America's great statements of moral identity. It is a celebration of the triumph of naïve, moral common sense over the petty, vain, greedy, and unjust social spectacles that Huck and Jim meet as they travel down the river. Both Crane and Twain were writing about freedom. Neither sought to define autonomy without coercion, or morality without guilt and shame.

COERCION AS A MORAL ISSUE

As we saw in chapter 8, ordinary definitions of coercion tend to treat it as the negation of autonomy; if autonomy connotes free space, privacy, a room of one's own, then coercion connotes constriction, binding, being boxed in. These ordinary language connotations inevitably cast coercion in a bad light and thus can be misleading ethically and philosophically.

When we perceive that one person's will is being bent by the force of another's and judge it a good thing, we tend to say that it's not "really" coercion. On the other hand, when we do not approve of a power relationship between two people, we label it "coercive," as if that alone were enough to condemn it morally.

Coercion is fast on its way to becoming one of the negative words in our social vocabulary that possesses a magic power of moral disapprobation by its mere utterance. *Murder, rape, incest, bigot, prejudice, chauvinism, paternalism*, and *harassment* are a few of the other words on that list. In no way can one defend a woman's right to abortion if one accepts the word *murder* as a description of the termination of pregnancy. A proper defense demands a rejection of the word *murder* to characterize the action.

When *coercion* is put into this category of self-condemning words, it is taken out of the flow of conversation, the exchange of good reasons, that should mark civic and moral discourse. It permits no give-and-take; it is a conversation-stopper, like pointing out that euthanasia is something the Nazis approved of and practiced. How can one continue the argument past this point without defending the indefensible?

When we grow accustomed to vetoing public policies and social practices that impinge upon autonomy simply by labeling them coercive, our
civic discourse suffers. When public debate no longer demands argument,
reason, and justification but merely the exchange of self-condemning words,
the habits and skills of argument will atrophy like unused muscles. We
will eventually lose the analytic abilities necessary to examine, reject, or
see what lies beneath a label. This atrophy must not be permitted with a
concept like coercion that is so critical to our social structure.

By labeling something "coercion" and thereby invoking the negative
moral force inherent in the word—rather than examining the underlying
reasons why an act may or may not be ethically justified—proponents of
both right- and left-wing policies can avoid facing basic assumptions and
practices that they would rather leave unexamined. Right-wing ranchers
who oppose environmental laws would prefer to brand federal efforts to
enforce the law as coercive rather than publicly admit that their own
short-term needs take precedence over the long-term public interest. Left-
wing advocates routinely resist as coercive and disrespectful any public
policies intended to change the self-destructive behavior of the "power-
less"—whether it be long-term contraception for adolescents or financial
incentives to break the cycle of welfare dependence. Coercion is said to
be inherent in such policies because of the pervasive powerlessness of
these people. So preoccupied are the advocates with not committing the
sin of "blaming the victim" that they often overemphasize the passivity
and helplessness of the very people whose interests they are trying to
serve. They thereby perpetuate passivity and encourage a victim mentality
instead of promoting the personal sense of responsibility that is essential
to empower people authentically and aid them in turning their own
lives around.

A blanket rejection of anything "coercive" or "paternalistic" often blinds
the defenders of autonomy and rights to the merits of innovative responses
to social problems. Sometimes these responses take the form of laws and
government regulations, but at other times they bubble up from grassroots
initiatives in the sphere of civil society. Sometimes the two sources work
in tandem. For example, the most effective efforts to reduce automobile
fatalities involving drunken driving are those that combine tough laws
and enforcement with concerted campaigns in schools and local communities for public education, peer pressure, and support programs, such as

designated-driver arrangements and late-night volunteer transportation programs for teenagers.

This is but one example of the link between the success of public policies originating in the sphere of the state and the health of institutions in the sphere of civil society. This link is stressed by sociologist Robert Putnam and others.[10] Government initiatives as varied as public health measures to control the spread of AIDS or sexually transmitted disease, job training programs, the promotion of business enterprise in minority communities all depend for their success on an infrastructure of "social capital"; that is, they depend on an underlying network of support groups, civic organizations, and voluntary organizations that help give needy individuals both the motivation and the human resources necessary to take advantage of these programs and to successfully modify their behavior.

A Framework for the Ethical Evaluation of Coercion

The capacity for moral debate and analysis concerning coercion must be rehabilitated in American civic discourse. We suggest the following framework of guidelines, principles, and concepts to promote that rehabilitation.

Coercion, in and of itself, is ethically neutral. Coercion is always a means to an end; it is neither intrinsically right nor wrong. To be coercive, an act need not harm or disadvantage the person being coerced—contrary to what Robert Nozick and Joseph Raz, among many other liberal and libertarian philosophers, maintain.[11] Carrots are as coercive as sticks. The ethical justification of coercion hinges on its relation to other values, and to a factual analysis that determines whether coercion promotes or impedes those values.

Coercion must be judged in a particular context. It is not coercion as such that we should ethically evaluate, but particular instances or acts of coercion under specific circumstances. In other words, the ethical justification of coercion must be contextual; it cannot be justified or condemned in the abstract, only in a particular setting and situation. Coercion functions differently in different spheres of life, and the conditions for justifying it will change as the arena of conduct changes. Justifying coercion in the relationship between a policeman or government official and a private citizen is not the same, for example, as justifying coercion in the relationship between an employer and an employee, or between friends, siblings, or spouses, or between a parent and a teenager. Coercion in different spheres has the same general properties—it is always an exercise of power or influence that alters individual behavior. But the motives, means, and circumstances of coercion will differ in different contexts. The values at stake will differ, and the impact of coercion on the relationship between the individuals over time will vary.

One reason why we may be willing to put up with types of coercion between friends or family members that we would not tolerate with government officials is that in the former situations there are ongoing relationships that temper coercion and protect against its excess or abuse, whereas no such personal relationships are present with coercive governmental authority. Therefore, state coercion is more subject to abuse, and stricter controls and limits on it are called for.

Three spheres of society must be distinguished when considering the ethical justification of coercion. The dividing lines among these spheres are not always bright and sharp, and the ways in which they can affect one another is usually very significant for the workings of social policies and efforts to change individual behavior. Nonetheless, they can be distinguished functionally and analytically. These sectors are the state, civil society, and the family.

The *state* is the locus of collective sovereign power and authority in a society. It is the form of association that has the task of setting forth the conditions for all the other forms of association; it sets the rules for setting the rules, and often goes on to establish particular rules in many areas of social life as well. The state enjoys what Max Weber referred to as a monopoly on the legitimate use of physical force in a geographic territory. The word *legitimate* is the key to this definition. Violence and physical coercion may certainly be employed by social organizations subsumed under the authority of the state, but they are by definition criminal activities. States come into existence only when private armies are brought under control, and when private individuals can no longer claim the autonomous discretion to use violence in a rightful way. The institutional structure through which the sovereignty of the state is exercised is usually called the government or the regime, and the rules of the state are the laws.

Civil society is the sector of voluntary associations that stand midway between the state and the market. Civil society is the arena of organizations of shared purpose or belief—churches and clubs, professional groups and charitable societies, universities and cultural bodies. Civil organizations are not authorized to make rules for other groups in the civil society, but they are usually given sufficient leeway by the state to make rules governing their own internal life. They mobilize and motivate individuals in a mixed and complex fashion—partly by a sense of moral conviction, partly by a sense of rational advantage, partly by a desire for a community of like-minded people, and partly for the experience of acting in concert with others in practical problem-solving and a sense of mutual need and common purpose.

Within civil society is a special sector called the *market*. It is the sector of society that organizes the fundamental human activities of making a living—production, consumption, and exchange. If the prime function of the state is rule (or rule making), the prime function of the market is to mobilize and organize the human effort that turns natural objects into objects for human use and consumption. The state motivates human activity and gives it a certain shape, channeling it in certain directions: negatively, through the threat of punishment, and positively, through a rational sense of justice or rightness and an emotional sense of patriotism. The market operates through calculations of rational self-interest and the profit motive. It is the most rationalistic and libertarian zone of society.

Civil society is the realm of community, mutual aid, and solidarity. Markets have entrepreneurs—literally givers and takers. They stay in relationship only as long as each individual realizes his or her own purposes in the relationship. States have rulers and subjects, with relationships hierarchically established, even if (as in democratic governments) only temporarily. These relationships endure as long as justice and order are served. Civil society is made up of citizens properly so called, whose relationships are equal and reciprocal. They may serve the ends of both justice and self-interest, but the distinctive force that holds civic relationships together is the satisfaction of some public or shared purpose: not what's in it for me, but what's in it for us; or more precisely, not what's in it for me-as-a-person-separate-from-others, but what's in it for me-as-a-person-in-relationship-with-others; what's in it for me as a part of us.

The *family* is the basic unit of biological production and social reproduction in a society. Its forms of organization and its governing norms vary considerably from one society to another and from one historical period to another, but its basic functions are dictated by the evolutionary nature of human beings—our developmentally premature birth, our prolonged period of physical and social dependence, our capacity for symbolic thought and communication, and our relative plasticity and behavioral dependence on social learning. Families are the spaces in which the profound intimacy of human sexuality, childhood, and parenting is played out. They are also the form of social organization through which is expressed what some paleontologists believe is the advantageous evolutionary propensity of *Homo sapiens* to form cooperative and stable mixed gender pairings.[12]

Coercion must be judged by its details. Agents of coercion set background conditions against which individuals must define their motivation and choose a course of action. An "agent" can be either a person or an institution, a set of rules, or a cultural atmosphere. In order to coerce his victim to part with his wallet, a mugger takes a number of steps to set up the background conditions for that behavior. He displays the weapon; he convinces the victim he is prepared to use it, by his menacing demeanor or tone of voice. In a similar way, for rules and mores to have a coercive power, they must set up the background conditions that will motivate socially valued behavior.

In evaluating a particular instance of coercion, then, the agent of coercion must be identified. Once that is done, the agent's motives for coercion must be assessed. Clearly, this is more straightforward in the case of individuals who coerce than it is in cases of coercion stemming from institutional or cultural conditions. The ethical assessment of coercion is not different in kind from the ethical assessment of other forms of action. Coercion driven by greed, hatred, selfishness, and the desire to dominate the other is never justifiable.

In addition to the motives behind coercion, the outcomes of coercion are significant for ethical analysis. Coercion always involves an implicit comparison of two different courses of action: the action that results due to the coercion, and the action that would have resulted if the coercion had not taken place. So the outcomes must be evaluated in both absolute and relative terms. Did the action that actually took place have ethically good consequences? Was it better than what the person would have done anyway? When coercion produces an evil act, it cannot be justified. It is never justified to coerce someone into committing murder; or into condemning one child to die so that another can be saved, the unspeakable circumstance of coercion depicted in William Styron's novel *Sophie's*

Choice.[13] Moreover, coercion should produce a better outcome than the autonomous choice would have. If it does not, then the coercion was otiose and therefore unjustifiable.

The effects of coercion on the person being coerced, and not just on other people or society as a whole, must also be considered. Coercion that makes a trivial difference in the behavior of the person is not as ethically troubling as that which causes the person to lose or forgo something important. Traffic laws that dictate driving on the right side of the road rather than the left are coercive in a trivial way; Jim Crow or apartheid laws that force black children into inferior schools are serious. The former hardly needs ethical justification at all; the important thing is that everyone follow the same rule. The latter can never find reasons strong enough to justify them. No appeal to social utility, traditional morality, or social order is compelling enough to overcome the harmful effects of this kind of coercion on the persons coerced.

Coercion exists along a spectrum of means. Finally, the means utilized to coerce are ethically significant. Coercion, it is often said, is not a single type of influence but a spectrum of influences ranging from mild to strong, from a pole of reason to a pole of emotion. Rational persuasion stands at one end of this spectrum, and threat of torture or violent death stands at the other. Some would speak of "coercion" only at the most threatening and emotion-laden end of the spectrum, but we prefer to define coercion as covering the entire range. Persuading, enticing, inducing, cajoling, pleading, tempting, seducing, admonishing, arm twisting, offering, threatening, frightening, indoctrinating, "brainwashing"—the list of terms goes on, and its length and diversity suggest that our everyday language must equip us to make rather fine distinctions. The characteristics of snow are important to Inuits for survival in their environment, and it is said that their language contains an extraordinary number of words for the different types of snow. Coercion is as omnipresent and diverse in the modern technological society as the snows in Greenland.

Moral evaluation requires these distinctions, but the metaphors of coercion are often imprecise. To place reason at one end and emotion at the other, and then to say that the farther one moves toward emotion, the less ethically justifiable influence becomes, is to embrace a false psychology and an insupportable morality. This is done by those, most famously John Stuart Mill in *On Liberty*,[14] who find persuasion or appeals to reason acceptable in attempting to change a person's behavior, but not more emotionally oriented appeals. The spectrum of coercion must be redrawn so that it no longer sets up a dualism between reason and emotion. We must avoid the old philosophical hierarchy of the mind in which reason represents the true or "higher" self compared with the "lower" passions or emotions. Instead, the proper polarity is to contrast motivation based on the social emotions with motivation based on purely primitive emotions. Both may operate through the reasoning and executive functions of the self.

Toward the first pole, we have motivation that involves appeals to principled convictions and self-respect reinforced by guilt, shame, and pride. At the other pole are punitive threats that tap into self-preservative fear and coercive emotional appeals that play upon anger, rage, jealousy, and lust. Somewhere in the middle we have hybrid feelings such as guilty fear or shame colored by anger.

Coercion near the pole of moral conviction, conscience, and the social emotions is more readily justified than coercion at the other end: not because the more primitive emotions are somehow less truly a part of the self, or are less fully human—we do not find these considerations particularly clarifying or convincing—but for two different reasons. First, coercion through the social emotions is a less direct assault on freedom and responsible agency than coercion through the primitive emotions; and second, it is less open to unethical abuse by agents of coercion for selfish or maleficent ends. Incentives appealing to self-esteem and self-betterment, such as job training or reproductive counseling programs, are more likely to promote responsible behavior than to undermine it. They are also more likely to be used for the good of the person subjected to them and are less likely to be abused. Incentives that intimidate, that use power to exploit and perpetuate its victims' weakness, and that appeal to greed are examples of the abuse of coercion.

Measures that exploit public disclosure and shaming are often coercive in a morally legitimate way. They induce better conduct by those persons, fully capable of acting responsibly, whom the shelter of anonymity has allowed to be morally careless. An example of coercion in such a case is the publishing of the names of parking scofflaws in the local newspapers. There is no question that appeals to shame represent abridgments of personal autonomy in particular instances. But they do not undermine the person's capacity for socially responsible conduct in the future. And they do not dehumanize or demoralize the person being coerced. On the contrary, by shaming someone, you publicly acknowledge his humanity and moral personality. Shame links the person to the community of which she is a part; even though the normal psychological response to shame is to withdraw from public view, shame in essence is less an emotion of separation than an affirmation of membership in a fellowship of people whose judgment matters to one's self-esteem.

Appeals to fear, anger, and envy are more easily abused, especially in the political realm, and coercion based on them is more likely to dehumanize those who are subject to it than to make them into responsible moral agents. Such coercive means should be used only in those cases where appeals to social emotions would not be effective. The sociopath is the prime example. Very young children are also examples, although for obviously different reasons. When it is developmentally appropriate, or when the social stakes are very high, primitive coercion may be justified. Otherwise, our ethical preference tilts toward coercion that makes use of what Abraham Lincoln called "the better angels of our nature": our conscience and the normal human desire to be a "good" person.

Justifying Coercion: Some Examples and Conclusions

Today, frustrated by real and perceived threats to the social order, many states and local communities are examining coercive measures to reinforce standards of social behavior. We have chosen two examples for more extended discussion in order to illustrate how the ethical assessment of coercion presented in this chapter can be applied. In the next chapter we will discuss more fully the instructive example of the deinstitutionalization and treatment of the mentally ill. These cases all illustrate the difficulty of choosing between social interests and individual rights.

Cocaine Use by Pregnant Women

Beginning in 1989 the Medical University of South Carolina in Charleston (MUSC), in cooperation with city and state law enforcement officials, carried out a program in which pregnant women in MUSC's prenatal clinic were tested for cocaine use. Those who tested positive were required to undergo mandatory drug and prenatal treatment, or their records would be turned over to the police. By 1994, forty-two women had been arrested during this period and several went to jail. The program was suspended when a class-action lawsuit charging racial discrimination was filed and when the Department of Health and Human Services threatened to cut off federal funds to the medical center.

Behavior control of pregnant women is one of the most highly charged areas of our society where autonomy and coercion collide. The cocaine screening and treatment program in South Carolina responded to the devastating physical and developmental disabilities that can be inflicted on an unborn child by its mother's use of crack cocaine.

The legal status of this issue is complex: there is no law in any state that specifically makes it a crime for a pregnant woman to harm her fetus by using harmful drugs, and yet more than 200 women have in fact been prosecuted for using illicit drugs or alcohol (which is every bit as harmful to the baby as cocaine) during pregnancy. Of course, coercion of this kind falls exclusively on women, and smacks of the notion that a pregnant woman may, while eating for two, have the rights of less than one.

Pregnancy is certainly a circumstance of special dependency and special responsibility. Most women understand this rationally and feel it spontaneously. They identify with their child-to-be and intuitively seek to ensure its well-being. Most women freely conform their behavior to the requirements of pregnancy. But it seems the more we learn about fetal development, the more we extend the range of proscribed behaviors and the more onerous these responsibilities become for all pregnant women.

Crack addicts are a special case. These women are often incapable of controlling their appetites for the drug short of miserable self-abuse and endangerment. Their drug dependence imposes a cruel restriction on their autonomy, even though they may desire to remain drug free during their pregnancy, knowing as well as anyone else what harm might be done to their baby.

The South Carolina program is a kind of middle ground between medical care and law enforcement, and thus it crosses the boundaries between the state and civil society. It also involves the relationship between a mother and her unborn baby and so enters the sphere of the family. Coercion here could be seen as a compensation for the loss of the normal capacity of self-control, if we assume that counseling and the threat of prison will have the desired motivating effect on most mothers.

Behavior modification achieved without the threat of criminal penalty, of course, would be preferable. A program that operated via such intervention and counseling would stay within the moral sphere of the doctor-patient relationship. The control and coercion inherent in rigorous counseling and twelve-step programs exploit a woman's natural desire to be a good mother and to protect her baby—rather than mobilize her primitive desire to avoid punishment.

Indeed, what ultimately led the U.S. Supreme Court to reject the MUSC program was the fact that it functioned more as an arm of law enforcement than as health care. It was more concerned with gathering evidence that could be used to prosecute women than it was with changing the women's behavior during pregnancy and improving the health outcomes for their babies. In the early 1990s, ten women who had been arrested due to the program brought suit. They lost a jury trial, appealed, and eventually the case went to the Supreme Court, which held that the MUSC program constituted a violation of women's constitutional rights under the Fourth Amendment as an unreasonable search because the women did not consent to the drug tests.[15]

We believe that this "softer" approach would have been more defensible ethically than what MUSC actually did. But the softer approach does not work in many cases. Coercion in some form is then justifiable to address the harm done to newborns by substance abuse. Doctors and hospitals cannot simply turn a blind eye to high-risk behavior when they detect it. Nor do women have a right to have them do so. Not even the right to obtain an abortion gives a woman the right to knowingly harm her fetus if she has decided to carry it to term; Roe v. Wade was not meant to signal the demise of all parental responsibilities during pregnancy.

Parental Liability for Juvenile Crimes

In January 1995 the small town of Silverton, Oregon, passed an ordinance that makes parents legally responsible when their minor children commit crimes. Penalties include a fine up to $1,000, paying restitution for damage done by the child, and mandatory parenting classes. A state law based on the Silverton ordinance has been passed by the Oregon legislature, and similar measures are under consideration in hundreds of cities around the country.

The Oregon parental responsibility law is an instance of coercion that we do not support. Although parents are surely morally responsible for any of their own behavior that affects their children, it is not at all clear that they are responsible for the behavior of their children that harms others. It is manifestly unfair to punish someone for something over which she has no control. Still, the question remains: how much can parents do to control the activities of their kids? Silverton city councilwoman Barbara Dahlum believes that parents can do more than they think and more than they are doing now: "Too many times I've heard parents say they can't do anything about their problem child—and this may be a kid who is only 7 years old. People have to be responsible for their kids. I would judge this law a success if it forces parents to get more involved in their children's lives."[16]

Still, in any given case, determining how much a parent could reasonably do, especially with teenagers, is difficult, and the courts are an ineffective instrument for such determinations. Even some of the supporters of the law in Silverton, like Dahlum, doubt that it would work in larger cities or more diverse communities.

Moreover, it is not the government that should be the primary organizing force that encourages "parents to get more involved in their children's lives." That force should more appropriately come from the realm of civil society. Making parents financially responsible for the damage their children do is reasonable; there is long-standing legal precedent for this in civil law, and it does not require new legislation like these so-called parental responsibility laws.

Forcing the parents of wayward youngsters into parenting-skill classes strikes us as a wrongheaded response, gratuitously humiliating where it is least needed and unlikely to work where it is most needed. For parents of children who are truly out of control, other resources and support services are required; that is a problem well beyond the reach of "parenting skills"— a term that itself displays naïveté about what can and cannot be taught.

We oppose such laws because they are an example of misplaced and overly intrusive governmental coercion. They are likely to be subject to arbitrary and selective enforcement. They are unlikely to have any long-term effect on the juvenile crime rate. And they will leave the bitter taste of unfairness in the mouths of those parents who are coerced by them. Good parenting emerges from positive values and relationships within a family, not from fear of legal punishment. Parental deficiencies and apathy are problems that need to be dealt with by the organizations in the civil society: churches, community organizations, schools, and civic groups.

When such deficiencies cross the border into abuse and neglect, we will label them as crimes, and only then will the state be the proper agent of control.

Coercion by the state must be subject to the tightest controls utilizing the narrowest grounds of ethical justification. State coercion is more likely to be punitive and based on the primitive emotion of fear of punishment than coercion in other spheres. The power of the state vis-à-vis the individual is always of moral moment. In the market, civil society, and the family, the ethical limits on coercion, and the protections of autonomy, need not be so stringent. The state is always available as an arena of appeal when coercion in other spheres fails.

We can afford to limit coercion by the state when other types of coercion are available and effective in other social spheres. When the mores of the family and the civil community do most of the work of maintaining social order, the coercive power of the state can be minimal. It is the anomic and disintegrated civil society—the so-called "mass society" of extreme individualism with social estrangement—that most readily succumbs to the rise of totalitarian state power.

On the other hand, because the purpose of civil and familial institutions is to foster socially responsible conduct, their methods of coercion will be practically and ethically limited—made obsolete by their own success. The goals of parental coercion must extend beyond the short-term protection of the child's best interests; the parent is charged with the responsibility of encouraging the emergence of a moral person and a good citizen. Coercion, therefore, cannot be a tool of short-term parental convenience. Parental influence and the careful use of coercion must be works of love in the hard and serious activity of living together in a family while rearing the young to a point of moral and social independence.

Similarly, the use of coercion among friends engaged in civic activities and relationships must be guided by the character and purposes of those relationships themselves. Justified coercion is never primarily about maintaining power, although it always involves the use of power. It is about maintaining functioning relationships of mutual obligation and responsibility.

In summary, coercion must be approached as something to be evaluated, not as something that is automatically wrong. Ethical analysis is necessary to evaluate the rightness or wrongness of any specific use of coercion. Such analysis must examine all of the elements of coercion, including the agent of coercion, the agent's motives, the consequences of coercion, and the psychological means used to achieve the behavioral objectives of the coercion.

Understood in these ways, coercion does not carry with it some hidden ideological agenda; it is not always the tool of the right or the enemy of the left or vice versa (as the neoconservatives and free-market libertarians of today would have us believe). It must be morally weighed in a pragmatic and nonideological spirit.

Finally, coercion is antithetical to autonomy only in particular instances and in regard to particular actions. In a broader sense, autonomy as a possibility in the real everyday lives of individuals depends upon the social control that coercion brings about. Autonomy requires limiting conditions as much as it requires enabling conditions. When autonomy must be limited by morally justified coercion, it cannot happen on autonomy's own terms; a richer vision of freedom and the human good than autonomy provides is required.

10

Autonomy Gone Bonkers: The Mentally Impaired

Not every defeat of authority is a gain for individual freedom, nor every judicial rescue of a convict a victory for liberty.

—JUSTICE ROBERT JACKSON,
"The Task of Maintaining Our Liberties"

THROUGHOUT THIS BOOK we have tried to show how the value of autonomy influences public policy as well as ethics in everyday life. At this point it may be helpful to focus on a practical case of autonomy theory gone awry. We now propose to look at two areas of social policy in detail to trace the perversion of autonomy in modern life. Many such case studies suggest themselves as possibilities for examination: the spread of AIDS, teenage pregnancy, drug and alcohol abuse, physician-assisted suicide and euthanasia, and welfare reform. We have chosen the story of the deinstitutionalized homeless, and the balancing story of psychological exculpation in the law. Here we can see directly how a wrongheaded emphasis on autonomy can lead to wrongheaded policies with disastrous social consequences.

Two aspects of current debates about mental impairment have led to opposite—and equally ludicrous—conclusions:

First, the homeless mentally ill—despite the obvious limitations of their judgment and autonomy—have been granted full responsibility for their lives and their treatment. In the clinical setting, we are gradually eliminating the population of the mentally impaired. Here we have a nonautonomous population granted full responsibility for their lives: responsibility without autonomy.

Second, in the courts of criminal law, we have extended the possibility of exculpability to a point where almost anyone may be perceived as mentally impaired. In the setting of social justice, we are gradually eliminating the population of the normal. Here we have the fully autonomous people freed from accountability: autonomy without responsibility.

THE HOMELESS MENTALLY ILL: RESPONSIBILITY WITHOUT AUTONOMY

The problem of "homelessness" presents a particularly clear example of what can happen when we press the concept of autonomy to a point of craziness. Most of us are familiar with the homeless mentally ill through our everyday contact with them in the streets of our cities. Theirs is a case that has been carefully studied and has a documented history. Three superbly researched but quite different works have cut through the miasma of political cant and propaganda and have shed the light of data and reason on this national disgrace. We are indebted to them and have drawn on them extensively.

The first of these works is Dr. E. Fuller Torrey's passionate and compassionate *Nowhere to Go: The Tragic Odyssey of the Homeless Mentally Ill*.[1] It is an indictment of the current state of affairs and the historic actions that brought them into being. Torrey sees homelessness as a product of calculated public policy—specifically the policy of deinstitutionalization, which he characterizes as "the dumping of the unwitting mentally ill into unwilling communities": Torrey brings to this problem the firsthand knowledge of a physician who understands only too well the nightmare conditions of severe mental illness. There is no romanticizing here.

The second book is by the distinguished liberal sociologist Christopher Jencks and is simply titled *The Homeless*.[2] With the precision of a surgeon and the dispassion and objectivity of a mathematician, Jencks attacks the mythology of homelessness, strips it of its political rhetoric, and exposes how the problem was created and maintained through the irresponsibility of reformers presumably acting to protect the rights and autonomy of the mentally ill.

Finally, a third superb source is Nancy Rhoden's "The Limits of Liberty: Deinstitutionalization, Homelessness, and Libertarian Theory" published in the *Emory Law Journal*.[3] Rhoden demonstrates how moral arguments once cast in terms of rights can be quickly translated into legislative and litigative principles that will then dictate and constrain all future policies.

How Many Homeless Are There, and How Many Are Mentally Ill?

Like spontaneous combustion, the homeless population seemed to emerge as if self-created. It was not. The size of the population then seemed to expand to startling and unpredictable size. It did not. The magnitude of the problem has been subject to the politics of reform and the ethics (or lack thereof) of advocacy. In 1984, as respectable an organization as the American Psychiatric Association included the following passage in the report of their Task Force on Homelessness: "Based on information received from more than 100 agencies and organizations in 25 cities and states, Hombs and Snyder (1982) estimated that there were as many as 2½ million homeless in the United States in 1980 and projected that the homeless populations could be as many as 3 million in 1983."[4]

Such estimates, the authors suggest, are "often advanced because of their shock value." Nonetheless they took these figures seriously and dismissed statistics proposed by the U.S. Department of Housing and Urban Development (HUD), which were consistently far smaller. By 1984 HUD had settled on an estimate of the homeless population at between 250,000 and 350,000. This estimate turned out to be accurate. Writing in 1994, Jencks concluded: "Any figure between 300,000 and 400,000 would be easy to defend. Estimates above 500,000 are considerably harder to reconcile with the available evidence."[5]

Who are these social statisticians, Snyder and Hombs, whose data were given such universal credibility, whose figures were lent respectability by the American Psychiatric Association? And how did they derive their figures? Mitch Snyder and Mary Ellen Hombs were political activists who coined the name *homeless* (thereby erroneously suggesting that the central problem was a matter of real estate rather than mental health). They were the leaders of the crusade identified with the Community for Creative Non-Violence. Where did they get their data? They made phone calls and came up with numbers that Snyder later admitted on *Nightline* had "no meaning, no value."[6]

We need not speculate about Snyder's motives—he revealed them. He had no idea what the correct number was; he knew that figures in the millions would command more attention than figures in the thousands, lending weight to his movement. Truth was irrelevant for political purposes. Why would politicians, social commentators, the press, and academia circulate the self-serving figures of advocates and activists rather than the carefully documented estimates of the government? The answer again must be drawn from the matrix of the time, the political climate of the 1970s and 1980s.

The egalitarianism and individualism of our heritage have always been accompanied by distrust of authority, and of government in particular. Since the mid-1960s, fed by the deceits and betrayals of the Vietnam war and the calumny of Watergate, healthy skepticism became raging distrust. The antiauthoritarianism of our time makes all data from the government suspect, just as the romantic individualism of our day allows us to abandon judgment and discrimination when dealing with the "data" of the reformer in his battle against the "powers that be." Nonetheless, detailed corroboration confirms that HUD was correct in its numbers, and Mitch Snyder wrong.

What percentage of the "homeless" are suffering from mental illness? The statistical data is not sufficient to be exact, but we can make reasonable estimates. The statistics vary depending on how one defines "mentally ill." The bias of the interviewer influences responses too, because definitions of mental illness are fuzzy and subjective. In any case, the estimates now run from 25 to 60 percent in most of the major cities. Most experts have settled on a figure somewhere between 35 and 40 percent. This figure refers to the seriously mentally ill (schizophrenic patients, for the most part) and does not include alcoholics or drug addicts. If one were to extend the definitions beyond the seriously mentally ill, to include the drug-addicted, the alcoholic, and the "mildly mentally ill," one would clearly be dealing with most of the adult homeless, something on the order of 200,000 to 300,000 people.

How Did They Get There? Deinstitutionalization
Christopher Jencks states: "As far as I can tell, the spread of homelessness among single adults was a by-product of five related changes: the elimination of involuntary commitment, the eviction of mental hospital patients who had nowhere to go, the advent of crack, increases in long-term joblessness, and political restrictions on the creation of flop houses. Among families, three factors appear to have been important: the spread of single motherhood, the erosion of welfare patients' purchasing power, and perhaps crack."[7]

From the 1950s to the 1970s there was a rapid discharge of mentally ill patients from hospitals. From a high of close to 600,000 in 1955, we had reduced the population to 171,000 by 1976. The patients were, for the most part, emptied out of the hospitals and dumped onto the streets.

What were the forces behind this movement for deinstitutionalization? According to Dr. Norman Q. Brill:

> Massive discharging of mentally ill patients from state hospitals was in part motivated by human concerns and in part by fiscal, legal, territorial, and anti-establishment considerations. Promises were made that the impaired adaptation resulting from hospitalization would be reversed by community-based treatment programs which would also be capable of identifying and eliminating ideological factors. Exploitation of patients would be eliminated and their rights protected. Not only were these objectives not achieved, but in some instances deinstitutionalized patients were worse off—ending up in poorly run nursing homes, board and care homes, welfare hotels, and jails. Many of the homeless are found to be mentally ill and hospital beds have become increasingly less available. Not only have patients' rights to decent treatment been compromised but so have the rights of society that is now expected to accept and tolerate all sorts of deviant behavior.[8]

First and foremost were humane concerns. Certainly the conditions in large state mental institutions were deplorable. Insufficient funds were available, and insufficient attention was paid to the hapless creatures who were often committed to their care. Rhoden states: "Studies in the 1950s and 60s revealed that public mental hospitals rather than being therapeutic communities were vast dehumanizing warehouses whose neglected, ill fed, and abused inmates could, with little exaggeration, be counted among the living dead."[9]

The term "warehousing" was to become an important shibboleth of the reform movement, and rightly so. It accurately described the conditions where patients were relegated to institutions for dispositional purposes alone and were maintained there with minimal care. Under these conditions of neglect, the patients often deteriorated severely. But these conditions had long existed, and reformers in each new generation had pointed out—over and over again—the inadequacies of our attention to the severely mentally ill. What differed this time around was that the reformers found themselves in sympathy with an age that offered supportive reinforcement. This period saw the birth of what may be referred to as the romantic view of mental illness.

In 1961 Dr. Thomas Szasz published an immensely influential book called *The Myth of Mental Illness*.[10] A reform movement that had originally been started to assault the dangerous expansion of mental illness to include more and more aberrant behavior finally became a movement to eliminate the concept of mental illness altogether—hence the "myth." Szasz became a hero of both the libertarian right and the libertarian left, who shared antiauthoritarian, antiestablishment sentiments. They seized on the concept of "labeling" as a means of denying mental illness. Mental patients were not sick; they had simply been labeled as such by establishment physicians. Aberrant behavior was actually a form of diversity. The libertarians then proceeded to romanticize the mentally ill in a series of plays and movies. The mentally ill were depicted as heroic and poetic figures, forced into conformity by a world of vulgarians. Literary figures such as Tennessee Williams, Ken Kesey, and Peter Schaffer and unconventional figures in psychiatry such as R. D. Laing helped establish the romantic concept of mental illness. Its central thesis was that not only are the mentally ill not ill, they are the only truly inspired and liberated members of our society. The romanticizers conveniently ignored the true suffering that mental illness causes. The ridiculous cliché that only the insane are truly sane became accepted. If that statement ever seemed acceptable, it was in the 1960s, when our political policies, and the responses to them, seemed crazier than much that goes on in mental institutions. The cult movie *The King of Hearts* was the perfect testament for the times.

Szasz himself had no illusions about the price that would be paid if one eliminated belief in the objective reality of mental illness. An illness is an exculpatory excuse for behavior. Without illness, one is responsible for one's actions. At a meeting in Hawaii, where Willard Gaylin shared a podium with him, Szasz was pressed by a young psychiatrist in the audience as to what should happen to a schizophrenic patient of his who was antisocial and uncontrollable. "He should be sent to jail," Szasz angrily responded. Unbeknownst to most of his followers on the left, who pursued his theme without reading his text, Szasz's views were actually quite conservative, if not right-wing. He had no compunctions about maintaining law and order. He simply wanted it done by law and order people. He was a man committed to the concept of responsibility.

The romanticizing movement created the kind of environment in which a distinguished professor of constitutional law could feel free to argue, without embarrassment, for deinstitutionalization on the grounds of "diversity." The mentally ill would enrich the cultural landscape of our cities, he maintained, just as African Americans, Asians, and other "minority groups" had. He dismissed the "exile" of the mentally ill to hospitals and institutions as a form of apartheid. This distinguished professor has since moved from the quiet haven of his midwestern university to an east coast campus, where his views have changed. Many suspect that it was his exposure to the "enriched environment" of diversity on the east coast campus that changed his views. Here the cultural diversity he could enjoy now included pathetic elderly women rummaging through garbage pails for scraps of food and psychotic men defecating on the sidewalk. Or more charitably, it may be that the passage of time revealed the bankruptcy of the promise of deinstitutionalization even to one of its architects.

The model and language of the civil rights movement, born of racial injustice, was now being extended to other movements for "liberation." Women's groups and gay rights movements followed the pattern. "Rights" were further defined as special claims, which meant they could be extended to any deprived group needing special attention. Why not to the mentally ill? Rights movements of all sorts were on the march, and morality was always cast in rights talk. The sociology of the times supported it.

The brilliant sociologist Erving Goffman reinforced the new anti-institutional trends with his assault on all "total institutions," viewing them as, by definition, destructive environments. At one meeting he supported this view with the statement that the similarities between Andover or Groton, and Attica or Creedmoor State Hospital were far greater than the differences. Some wag pointed out that one was likely to meet a "classier" set of people at Andover than at Attica. At any rate, the stage was set for the mentally ill to be viewed as simply one more oppressed minority.

Under these circumstances there emerged a consanguinity between left and right, always a dangerous situation. The left-wing reformers, who were determined to deinstitutionalize on the assumption that they were serving patients' rights, were joined by conservatives, who were delighted at the opportunity to reduce state mental health costs, an area of expenditure they had never supported anyway. These institutions had always been underfunded, and now with the reduction of 60 to 80 percent of their population, most could simply be shut down. They embraced the reformist cause of deinstitutionalization with a vengeance—and the mentally ill were crushed in the process. Andrew Scull, from a left-wing radical perspective, popularized the opinion that economic savings were the primary motivations.[11]

Nonetheless, it would still have been difficult to dump three-fourths of the severely mentally ill into city streets without some ancillary support. The 1950s had seen the emergence of the first drugs that helped to manage and control the violent behavior of schizophrenic patients. Chlorpromazine entered the marketplace in 1954, the first of many antipsychotic drugs that, although not curing psychosis, made psychotic patients more tranquil and less destructive.

Medicated psychotics were less agitated and more tractable. Many rights advocates thought it perfectly safe to release them to the streets, forgetting that once out there, no supervision would be present to ensure they took their medication. The reformers, consistent with the conspiratorial mood of the times, saw even the emergence of the first reasonably successful psychotropic drugs as but another manipulative exploitation. They saw only the potential of the medications for "drugging a population into submission" rather than relieving them of some of their more horrible psychotic symptoms.

Only when one examines some of the deinstitutionalized patients who were given the "autonomy" to pursue their own idiosyncratic and diverse lives can one fully appreciate the horror of such libertarian generalizations.

Consider Timothy Waldrop, a victim of deinstitutionalization, who was twenty-four years old and who had been voted the friendliest boy in his high school graduating class. He had been treated for schizophrenia for several years. He was arrested for armed robbery and sentenced to five years in a Georgia state prison. In prison his antipsychotic medication was stopped. According to newspaper accounts, "a few days later Waldrop gouged out his left eye with his fingers." Despite resuming his medication, he then cut his scrotum with a razor and while in restraints "punctured his right eye with a fingernail, leaving himself totally blind."[12]

The Lawyers and Legislature Join In

In the 1960s a powerful push from psychiatry and its friends was instituted to revamp the care of the mentally ill. The magic touchstone of the movement was the concept of the community mental health center as an alternative to existing mental institutions. In 1963 Congress adopted an act than provided federal funding to develop and encourage the growth of community mental health centers. Remember that this movement marched under the banner of liberty and autonomy. The mentally ill were not really sick, they had only been labeled so, and under this label they were being deprived of their autonomous rights. As Rhoden describes it:

> The early advocates of deinstitutionalization harbored an idealized notion of "community" and tended to exaggerate the extent to which labeling a person mentally ill produces and perpetuated pathology. Consequently, they were overly optimistic in their assessment of the ability of released patients to survive, unaided, in society. . . . Many legal advocates of patients' rights shared these assumptions and coupled them with a skepticism, albeit often healthy, about psychiatric diagnosis and treatment. Therefore, they focused far more heavily on obtaining liberty for patients than on seeking services for them. Since judicial decrees can grant rights against government infringement of liberty far more easily than they can establish positive entitlements to care and services, the result was that mental patients obtained their liberty, but at the expense of the community care they so desperately needed?[13]

The tragic failure of the community mental health center movement is too complicated to be presented in detail here. The reasons for its failure are as multiple as the factions in our political spectrum. The one thing about which there is unanimity is that the movement was a total failure. Nonetheless, one must remember the hopes of its advocates: it would enhance liberty, remove the coercion and paternalism of bureaucracy and government, and allow patients on their own initiative (with the funding of the government) to form self-supporting, self-sustaining independent communities. The introduction of Medicaid in 1965 was a necessary condition to serve this movement. Medicaid does not cover treatment for the institutionalized mentally ill. But if such people live in residential homes or nursing homes, it pays for most of the care. This became a powerful incentive for states to cash in on the honey pot of Medicaid by transferring all of their patients out of the mental institutions—for which the states were financially responsible—into euphemistically named facilities that were federally fundable. The fiscal conservatives in state governments eventually saved taxpayers money with official neglect, which eventually became the substitute for care.

All this must be perceived in the context of the times. Very real progress was made during the 1960s and 1970s in securing human rights for oppressed minorities—all aided by the courts. "By the early 1970s most civil liberties lawyers endorsed Szasz's argument that we should lock up the mentally ill only if they broke the law. The Supreme Court encouraged such thinking throughout the 1970s. In 1975, for example the Court ruled in O'Connor versus Donaldson that mental illness alone was not sufficient justification for involuntary commitment. By the end of the 1970s almost every state had made it impossible to lock up patients for more than a few days unless they posed a clear danger to themselves or others."[14]

At the same time the courts, goaded by reformist lawyers, were unable to perceive the difference between mainstream civil rights issues and deinstitutionalization. Discrimination against racial minority groups is arbitrary and unjust. However, limiting the liberties and privileges of the mentally ill, at least to some extent, is a necessary response to the very real incapacity of these people to care for themselves. The arguments for rights of minorities such as African Americans and women had been moral assaults on bias and bigotry. What distinguishes black from white—the color of a person's skin—ought to have no moral significance in our society. People should be judged as individuals on the basis of their conduct, not as members of a group. Civil rights in this sense means nondiscrimination on the basis of morally irrelevant characteristics in the schools, in the workplace, and in public spaces. This understanding of the civil rights argument puts African Americans (and other minorities) in the position of asking not for special treatment but only for the ordinary dignity of citizenship. Civil rights allow people to be recognized as full and complete members of the moral and civic community.

The severely mentally ill are, however, a group *defined* by their common difficulties in coping. Their condition demands special consideration and special treatment. They require a distinctive moral response to their needs and limitations; they deserve it on the basis of decency and compassion. Recognizing their needs does not deny them respect as persons; on the contrary, it is society's failure to recognize their special needs and vulnerabilities that is dehumanizing to the mentally impaired. The severe schizophrenic ought not be treated as a normal autonomous individual. We do not turn over the management of his finances to him; we should not have turned over the more important responsibilities of his medical treatment. Membership in that group by definition consists of people who need help. It is neither patronizing nor an injustice to treat a deteriorated schizophrenic or a severely mentally retarded person with beneficence. As Jencks writes:

> Limiting the rights of the mentally ill on the grounds that they are too confused to know their own interests or to respect the rights of others led to many abuses. But the fact that a principle is often abused does not mean it is wrong. . . . The civil liberties lawyers . . . thought individual autonomy so important that they could hardly imagine patients who would be better off when other people told them what to do. They also identified so strongly with the oppressed that they could not take seriously the idea that releasing mentally ill patients from hospitals might make the rest of us worse off.[15]

But the courts were on a roll, and the reformers pressed even further. They first ruled that a mentally ill patient could not be institutionalized—regardless of how incapable he was of taking care of the rudiments of his own survival—without clear evidence that he would be harmful to himself or others. But that harmfulness could almost never be proved. The restrictive definitions of "dangerousness" given by most courts are astonishing. Eventually, a person could be institutionalized only if they actually committed an act of violence. And even this evidence may suffice for only a short hospitalization, after which the patient would have to commit another crime in order to be rehospitalized.

Commitment procedure was not the only problem that resulted from deinstitutionalization. For years various state courts had been finding that patients must not be "coerced" into taking any treatment against their will, including simple medication. Then in 1979 a federal judge in Massachusetts decreed that a patient has a right to refuse medication unless there is clear evidence of "a substantial likelihood of extreme violence, personal injury, or attempted suicide."[16] This means just what it says: a delusional patient has a right to refuse any medication, safe or otherwise, for the worst of reasons; for example, he is convinced that the penicillin offered to treat his suppurative, self-inflicted wound is really a poison.

Psychiatrists were now placed in the untenable position that they could not hospitalize a patient for his own interests unless he had first committed violence, and once he was in the hospital, they could not treat a patient who refused treatment without petitioning the courts for permission. Thus—ironically—the reformers had managed to legitimate a new form of "ware-housing." What else can one call confining someone to an institution without treatment? The paradox for psychiatrists became greater when the courts decided that any patient not receiving active treatment must be quickly discharged. So discharge them they did.

Where did all of these patients end up? The evidence is clear. The newly liberated population of deinstitutionalized patients was apportioned between the prisons and the streets. Thomas Szasz had his way—the mentally ill were liberated from the malevolent authority of psychiatry and placed under the tender ministrations of the criminal justice system. And the reformers had their way—the mental institutions were emptied, and mentally ill patients were granted their freedom to defecate, urinate, sleep, starve, freeze, murder, and be murdered in the streets of our larger cities. All in the name of autonomy.

The ethics of advocacy needs to be reexamined. The world of theory must confront the world of reality. Reality exists in the faces of the people in the streets. Fuller Torrey looked at those faces and shared his appalling experience with us. Here are two people, from his personal experience, who demonstrate the humane world that emerges when mental illness is treated as a myth, when beneficence is sacrificed to the illusion of autonomy.

> When I saw Mr. A I hardly recognized him. He had been sleeping in fields and abandoned barns for several months. His clothing and hygiene betrayed his chronic psychotic state. He agreed to meet me outside the District of Columbia line, saying that he could not go into the District because the FBI might pick him up. He believed

they had planted electrodes in his brain, which he heard as voices, so he had to be careful. He refused all offers of medication. I remembered him as one of the leaders of my graduating class at Princeton University, a young man with an obviously bright future.[17]

Mr. A suffers from acute schizophrenia. Without receiving any modern treatments, one-third of acute schizophrenia patients would go into spontaneous remission, one-third would never recover, and one-third would respond to care and supportive therapy. But this last third have to be getting the care. Modern drug therapy has increased the chances for remission and significantly enhanced our ability to control the symptoms that cause schizophrenic patients agonies and disorientation. In the past, psychiatrists often had to force the treatment, to the later gratitude of their recovered patients. But not anymore. Mr. A has been given the legal right to exercise his autonomy. He is now "free" to refuse all medication. Alas, he is not "free" to enter the District; if he does, the FBI might capture him and plant electrodes in his brain for the secrets and secret sins within him.

Consider one other case of autonomy gone bonkers:

A 29-year-old woman, arrested for breaking an antenna off a car, gave birth to a baby in a cell of the Erie County Holding Center, a county jail in Buffalo. Nobody, including the woman, was aware that she had been 8 months pregnant. She was known to be seriously psychotic, and at the time of the birth screamed loudly to the guards to get the "animal" out of her clothing. By the time the guards retrieved the baby it was dead. At the time the jail was estimated to be holding more seriously mentally ill persons, approximately 90, than was the psychiatric unit of the Erie County Medical Center.[18]

To treat the seriously mentally ill as though they had capacities to exercise normal levels of autonomy is an act of barbarism that can only represent either an incredible naïveté or a moral readiness to distort reality to serve a political agenda. One could argue that the social scientists and reformers were simply ignorant of the massive debilitation of severe mental illness. Yet many of the reformers, including Szasz, came out of the mental health programs; furthermore, there ought be an ethics of advocacy that requires such knowledge.

Jencks aptly summarizes the problem when he states, "The strongest argument for coercion is that we have an obligation to protect everyone's better self from the darker forces that sometimes rule them."[19]

When those darker forces are ruling people, they are not acting as free people would act. Friends and family are alerted to severe mental illness when they notice that their colleagues or loved ones are "not acting like themselves." The commonsense awareness of those who know and love them should be heard above the din of the advocates and the theorists. The mentally ill are *not* themselves. And they are not free. Henri Bergson recognized this when he stated: "We are free [and by implication *only* free] when our actions emanate from our total personality, when they express it, when they resemble it in the indefinable way a work of art sometimes does the artist."[20]

THE COERCION EXCUSE: AUTONOMY WITHOUT RESPONSIBILITY

If our current attitudes about the mentally ill represent the folly of giving someone autonomy when he lacks the capacity to exercise it, our attitudes about social transgression represent the opposite absurdity: allowing those who should acknowledge their autonomy and accept responsibility for what they do to use coercion as an excuse.

Modern psychology in the twentieth century has redefined the self. But the culture of autonomy has perversely misapplied most of psychology's lessons. What are those lessons?

- We are less autonomous (freely choosing) than we would like to believe. The individual in the present is beholden to—and often in the service of—his past. Early development counts.

- We are less rational than we would like to believe. Adult behavior is resistant to change. In many ingrained areas, emotional pressures are more likely to succeed than rational appeals. "Education" is unlikely to change fixed addictive behavior like cigarette smoking, alcohol and drug abuse, or irresponsible sexuality.

- The individual cannot be separated in his interests from the culture that cradled him and the society that sustains him. There is no autonomous (self-sustaining) individual. Press individual rights to the neglect of society, and you will end up destroying both.

Conservative libertarians never bought any of this "bleeding heart" psychology (any more than orthodox Marxists did). They were firm in their nineteenth-century view of the rugged individualist, now armed to the teeth, needing to defend himself against coercive government and anything else standing in his way. More moderate liberals have managed to accept the first lesson with a vengeance—accepting all sorts of exculpations for antisocial behavior. At the same time they totally ignore the last two lessons, as though these linked and inseparable components of a self could possibly be rent asunder.

As a result, the culture of autonomy has created a strange chimera as its ideal: a freestanding individual for whom privacy and autonomy are sacred virtues, independent of his community, with almost unbridled authority over his actions and with no responsibility for its consequences. It has created a society of rights without duties or obligations; of authority without responsibility.

The danger of determinism that is inherent in their own developmental theory was early apparent to psychoanalysts. By showing that present-day behavior is causally related to the past, psychoanalysts seemed to be heading toward an unconditional determinism that was anathema to them. Their very treatment methodologies required a responsible aspect of the ego and superego that could exercise control over destructive impulses from the id. They compromised by suggesting that although behavior might not be changeable through rational discourse alone, personal behavior might not operate entirely outside the realm of rational control. After all, even when an individual operates only on the primitive level of fear, if he knows that a terrifying punishment would ensue from acting on his antisocial impulses, he will generally control those impulses. Anticipating punishment is a process of the rational mind, not the emotions.

Psychoanalysts were capable of resolving the dilemma of determinism and accountability by exploiting the special moral conditions that adhere to the "sick role." Like all patients, the neurotic as well as the psychotic individual would not be held responsible for his "symptoms." Therapists retained accountability for behavior—and the compassionate and nonjudgmental aspects of the physician's role—by defining neurotic behavior as a sickness and therefore exempt from moral judgment. They were operating under the ethical rules of the special case, the patient.

However, the liberal community—in alliance with certain leaders of the psychoanalytic establishment—began to extend the sick model into all aspects of sociological and psychological behavior, to a point where no one could be held accountable for anything. The irrationality of this extension is best dramatized by what has been happening in our courts of law; the most important aspects of nonaccountability, however, may actually be appearing in the everyday social world around us.

With the decline of the power of a religious vision, modern culture abandoned the concept of absolute rules whose violations constituted sins. It began to approach questions of right and wrong almost exclusively from a sociological and psychological frame of reference. We judged an action by considering the events that led up to the conduct. Psychology contributed to a more compassionate and sophisticated understanding of transgression and to a more refined sense of justice, but the extension of sociological and psychological exculpation ultimately proves self-defeating as it becomes all-inclusive. Eventually this extension will lead to a moral relativism, in which everything goes, because no one can be held accountable for anything.

This slide to relativism is dangerous—and is not in fact dictated by the findings of modern psychology. Human beings are endowed with a freedom from instinctual fixations that demands that we make important decisions—and be accountable for them. We must make decisions despite the fact that rationality is mitigated by emotion. The principle is fully compatible with the truth that the cultural past is a factor in our decisions of the present. The law rightly demands of us some acknowledgment of self-control, some acknowledgment of responsibility for action. It cannot operate without these assumptions. It makes no moral sense without them. But well before the emergence of modern behavioral psychology, the code of justice had been forced to deal with the perversity of human conduct and the complexity of human motivation.

Since the sixteenth century the insane have been acknowledged to be unable to tell right from wrong. They have been exempted from standing trial for their crimes, while still not being exculpated for their actions. Only much later would the principle of being "not guilty by reason of insanity" be introduced. Introducing this principle created a category of less responsible individuals, the mentally ill. By the nineteenth century, the insanity defense had become increasingly common, but until very recent times one had to be flagrantly psychotic in order to be excused from culpability on the basis of insanity.

This humane principle of diminished responsibility is now firmly established in our system of justice. It recognizes that the insane person occupies a world of his own, is estranged from reality, distorted in his perceptions, incapable of judging right from wrong; he is often incapable of knowing who he is, let alone whom he is accosting. The insanity defense is intended to protect the insane person from accountability for actions over which he had no control.

To be in this state is to be "mentally ill" and a "mental patient." A mental patient is not held accountable for his illness; a mental patient is the victim of his illness, not its cause. By defining a small percentage of the population as mentally ill and therefore not responsible for their actions, we were able to preserve the principle of accountability for the vast majority of "normal" individuals.

The concept of *mens rea* (from Latin, "things of the mind") is also central to our legal system today. It allows us to modify our moral judgment of criminal conduct by considering emotional conditions far short of insanity. An understanding of the accused's state of mind and his intentions is now essential in judging his conduct. The presence of "extreme emotional disturbance," for example, is sufficient in some jurisdictions to reduce murder to the lesser charge of manslaughter. But the insanity defense goes further; it can exculpate even homicide.

The Insanity Defense

The insanity defense is a prime example—indeed, the original example—of the awareness that there must inevitably be some exceptions in a justice system that demands that each individual be accountable for his actions and pay a significant and proportional price for defiance of the state's laws.

Today this initially reasonable and decent principle is being extended to alarming proportions of the population, thereby attenuating its moral significance. We are now at a point where it threatens the very concepts of accountability and responsibility. Criminal defense lawyers, unconcerned with any notion of justice but devoted to a passion for acquittal, have seized on the developmental insights of psychiatry and psychoanalysis and extended them to a point where almost any action, no matter how heinous, how calculated, how premeditated, or how motivated, can be perceived as having some psychological or sociological exculpatory defense.

The following few examples selected out of—unfortunately—a large group of possibilities further demonstrate the trend that concerns us.

Colin Ferguson. On December 7, 1993, Colin Ferguson, a black Jamaican immigrant from an affluent island family, then living in Brooklyn, boarded the 5:33 P.M. commuter train to Hicksville, Long Island. Unlike the majority of the people on that train who were coming home *from* business, Ferguson was there *on* business, on a mission of his own, that required not a packed briefcase but a semi-automatic weapon and thirty-six rounds of ammunition. A half hour into the trip, Ferguson got up and randomly, indiscriminately, and cold-bloodedly emptied his gun into the men, women, and children who were his unfortunate fellow passengers. With thirty rounds of ammunition he managed to kill six people and wound nineteen others. God knows how many more would have been killed had he been able to get another clip into his gun. Fortunately, a courageous passenger, at risk of his life, tackled Ferguson as he was reloading.

Colin Ferguson seems to have been the answer to the late William Kunstler's prayers, the ideal "victim" for our time. According to an article in *Vanity Fair* of January 1995, Kunstler, a renowned defense attorney, had been looking for a client like Colin Ferguson his entire career. Almost joyously Kunstler announced, "This is a direct assault on white racism and I've never had that before. I've never been able to put experts on the stand to talk about the effects of white racism in America on black people." His colleague Ron Kuby said, "The more the white community fears African Americans the better" and introduced yet a new disease to the psychiatric lexicon of excuse from personal responsibility. Colin Ferguson, Kuby decided, was suffering from "black rage." What is black rage, you might ask? It turns out that it is a "malignant psychological state" from which black people suffer by virtue of living in a predominantly white racist society.

Never mind that most black Americans who live in a predominantly white racist society have not developed a strange psychological condition that drives them to mass murder. Never mind that Ferguson was *not* reared in a white racist society but enjoyed an affluent upbringing in Jamaica, where he was treated like a young prince, with limousines and chauffeurs to take him to his private school. The black rage defense did not help Colin Ferguson; he refused to use it, firing his ingenious lawyers and becoming his own defense lawyer. But the "black rage" defense lives on and has now entered into the criminal defense armamentarium of exculpating defenses. It is being introduced in many courtrooms to explain gratuitous black violence toward whites and even crimes against Latino/as, Indians, Koreans, and other assorted minority group members.

Rashid Baz. If black rage is sufficient to make one take a machine gun and mow down innocent people on a commuter train, "early Arab trauma" is an equally compelling mitigating motivation for the slaughter of the innocent. This exculpation has an authentic Freudian ring to it. In March 1994, Rashid Baz opened fire with an automatic weapon on a bus containing a group of yeshiva students. He had planted himself on the Brooklyn Bridge and ambushed a specific vehicle. In the limited time he had to fire at the moving vehicle, he only managed to kill one boy, sixteen-year-old Aaron Halberstam, but he did seriously wound three other students. The murder took place in broad daylight, in front of many witnesses, and was obviously preplanned. There seemed no obvious defense. Nonetheless, defense attorney Erik M. Sears, perhaps inspired by the ingenuity and imagination of colleagues like Kunstler and Kuby, suggested without apology that Rashid Baz was not truly a criminal but rather must be perceived as himself a "victim." After all, Baz had been raised for the first eighteen years of his life in Lebanon. Given that history, he could not possibly be legally responsible for the shootings. So psychologically scarred was he by the larger environment of his youth that he had no more control over or understanding of his own behavior "than a fire once lit understands why it's burning."

Realizing that no self-respecting jury is likely to confuse what a defense attorney says about his client's mental status with actuality, Sears sought the support of the "experts" in the field. Seek and ye shall find. With proper funds one has no difficulty finding expert witnesses prepared to discover in anyone some infantile trauma that may be used to exculpate any and all adult antisocial behavior. Sears could have utilized the antiquated World War I diagnosis of "shell shock," which is actually having a revival these days. Instead, he found an expert with a diagnosis of somewhat more cachet.

Dr. Nuha Abudabbeh, a Ph.D. in psychology with a clinical practice who hosts her own radio talk show, eschewed that old chestnut "shell shock" in favor of a newly coined clinical syndrome that she appropriately labeled "Early Arab trauma." What can we expect next? The religious, gender, and national psychic traumas remaining to be articulated suggest a veritable rainbow assortment of exciting and imaginative new psychological conditions to add color and creativity to the current diagnostic manual of psychiatric disorders.

But what of those poor criminals-*cum*-victims who can claim no special racial or cultural exculpation? We all have a developmental past, mommies and daddies, siblings and situations. From them, defense lawyers can always derive a plethora of *psychological* explanations, real or imagined. Because psychology by definition exists within the *perceptions* of the individual, one might say that reality is totally irrelevant. Most defense lawyers, however, would prefer not to tax the intelligence of a jury by inviting them to consider the perceived reality to which the accused was forced to respond. Why bother delving into these complexities of the human psyche when one can create an artificial set of historic grievances? Who would know? In most cases the victims who might contradict the revisionist history of the criminals are already conveniently dead.

Lorena Bobbitt. A case that achieved particular prominence for demonstrating the bizarre ability of a jury to find mitigation for mayhem is that of Lorena Bobbitt. On the night of June 23, 1993, Lorena Bobbitt selected a large carving knife from among her kitchen utensils, quietly entered her bedroom, where her husband lay peacefully asleep on their bed, and shortened his penis. Quick as a cat can wink its eye, Lorena Bobbitt became a feminist hero, having been declared a victim of chronic sexual abuse. Her lawyer put it bluntly: it was a question of "his penis versus her life." Expert witnesses were readily available to pronounce Lorena Bobbitt temporarily *insane*—whatever that means. As is customary in these cases, she was remanded to a mental hospital, which discharged her after a few months, because mental hospitals have no treatment facilities for sane individuals who are sent to them after their temporary states of insanity have vanished.

Erik and Lyle Menendez. The Menendez brothers are, of course, a different story. On August 20, 1989, Erik and Lyle Menendez, using a twelve-gauge shotgun, brutally shot and killed their mother and father as the old folks watched television in their own home. The boys did a good job. The father was shot at least five times, once at close range in the back of the head. The mother was shot ten times. She seemed to resist dying. Erik had to go out to get more ammunition. After reloading, they put the gun directly to her face to blast her one final time. The parents were both in their mid-forties; Erik was eighteen at the time, and Lyle twenty-one. After disposing of the shells and guns, the boys took in a good movie before reporting their tragic loss to the police.

The Menendez brothers, with all the money they had inherited from their parents, were capable of hiring a team of defense specialists unrivaled until the even more celebrated case of O. J. Simpson. Although a jury ultimately convicted them of murder, the brothers lavishly purchased psychologists, psychiatrists, and motivation authorities of all sorts, just as they purchased the Rolex watches, apartment condos, and luxury automobiles that were all part of their posthomicide spending spree.

Naturally the first step (as always) was to portray the boys as victims. A historic legacy of parental abuse—physical, psychological, and sexual— was set before the jury. A lifetime of contrary evidence, antisocial behavior, pathological lying, and general psychopathy on their part—always protected from the punishment of the law by indulgent and protective parents—was washed away by the lurid imaginations of the hired psychologists and psychiatrists.

Expert witnesses testified with absolute certitude all sorts of things of which psychiatrists in the normal everyday practice of psychiatry can never be certain. This testimony unblinkingly maintained that the boys were not lying about the details of their abuse; they could not have been lying, because they were essentially truth tellers by nature. Besides, "scientific evidence"—whose nature we have not been able to locate—shows that abused children undergo permanent changes in their "brain chemistry," which impels, even demands, such violent action.

In the same way that television sitcoms command a reality in the minds of many people that transcends the actuality of real events, the courtroom fantasies of psychological conjurers are now often afforded a greater validity by jurors than the actual evidence of real events.

PRESERVING RESPONSIBILITY

Obviously, if these high-profile cases were representative of typical transactions in the many courtrooms not covered by national media, the entire criminal justice system would be endangered by the establishment of a complete repertoire of excusing conditions for all human behavior. It will not happen—political realities will intervene. The greater danger may be in the cynicism, and contempt for the judicial system, that such outlandish defenses generate in the public mind.

The folly of all this exculpation was very early recognized. In 1760 an English solicitor general said:

> My Lords, in some sense, every crime proceeds from insanity. All cruelty, all brutality, all revenge, all injustice is insanity. There were philosophers in ancient times, who held this opinion. . . . My Lords, the opinion is right in philosophy but dangerous in judicature. It may have a useful and noble influence, to regulate the conduct of men; to control their important passions; to teach them that virtue is the perfection of reason, as reason itself is the perfection of human nature; but not to extenuate crimes, not to excuse those punishments which the law adjudges to be their due.[21]

One of the dangers of a runaway insanity defense—or a runaway inventory of psychological and social factors that are supposed to excuse people from individual accountability—is that it contributes to a dangerous counterreaction when its results defy everyday common sense. Although these most dramatic cases are admittedly few in number, their impact is often vast. These trials—now broadcast live on television—are precisely the kind of cases that gather public attention and incur public wrath. They then become conflated and confused with the public's already existing anxiety about law and order and contribute to the general feeling that "things are not working." The intellectual community—focusing on the limited number of such dramatic cases—has sadly neglected the disproportionate and devastating psychological effect they can have on ordinary people. The sense that justice is not prevailing, that the system is failing, is a terrifying and dangerous phenomenon. It encourages simplistic impulsive solutions and creates a mood of susceptibility to demagoguery, rhetoric, and quick-fix quackery. The shock of the O. J. Simpson verdict was nothing as compared with the dismay of the black-versus-white schism that it revealed and reinforced.

We must not overreact. There is always a tendency in this country to avoid complex moral issues by searching for simpler legal solutions. We will not improve our society by a restrictive, vindictive response derived from our internal fears. Thoughtful, unblinking debate about the complex nature of crime and accountability in an age of psychological sophistication is what is needed.

We must negotiate a new social contract that, although still respecting the individual, will more aggressively support and preserve the social structures and institutions necessary to sustain and define that individual. We must insist that culpability and responsibility be preserved and cherished, even in this world where sociological and psychological explanations for human conduct abound. The wife beater who "can't help it," who goes into "uncontrollable" rages, will have to answer why he never seems to lose control with his employer or a policeman. We must eschew both polarities. Human behavior must be understood as occupying some point along a continuum from psychic determinism to rational autonomy.

A human being who is so diminished that he is not constrained by shame or guilt will still respond to fear of punishment. But the fear must be real; the punishment sure, swift, and sufficiently severe. Even the lion will respond to the crack of the lion-tamer's whip. Still, we must not compromise our defining values for an incremental increase in security— America is not, and should not become, Singapore. The only whip here must be the fear of incarceration.

If, as some of these defenses claim, the human being is so depraved, so automatically driven by his developmental past, as to be beyond even the animal controls of fear, then the answer is still not exoneration. Such a person must not be returned to society. He must be locked away, for our sakes if not for his. The lion cannot be invited to lie down with the lamb. The peaceable kingdom is not yet at hand.

The conflicting attitudes presented here concerning the homeless and the criminal indicate the confusion that exists about the nature of human conduct. When it comes to autonomy, Americans have tried to have their cake and eat it too, and they are now gagging on it. We must build on our knowledge of the rules of conduct to construct a society that is stable, moral, and respectful of human interdependence. We must place the individual back into the community that sustains him. If we elevate the rights of the individual too far above his duties and responsibilities to family, community, and state, we will surely destroy him.

Only in human creatures is the self defined not merely by distinguishing it *from* others but relating it *to* at least some others. Our very "humanness" is a phenomenon of engagements and attachments. We survive in a network of relationships with other human beings. Each knot of individuality is bound to the next, creating the social fabric in which personhood has true existence. The isolated individual is an illusion. If we unravel the network of social contacts, the knots disappear.

II

Last Rights I: Decisions to Forgo Life-Sustaining Medical Treatment

We thank you for the blessing of family and friends, and
for the loving care which surrounds us on every side.
—*The Book of Common Prayer*

THE CULTURE OF autonomy in American life is like a large river with
many feeder streams. One of the most important sources of intellectual,
emotional, and moral support for the culture of autonomy during the last
three decades has come from the domain of health care.

Autonomy has been the rallying cry within health care for patients'
rights movements, particularly in the area of women's health. It has also
been at the center of our field of study, bioethics, where the principle of
autonomy or self-determination has been used most forcefully to bring
about changes in the way medical research on human beings is conducted
and also to change the assumptions and expectations underlying the physician-patient relationship.

Moreover, if our time will be remembered for anything distinctive it
surely will be our preoccupation with health, the body, and all things
biological, from the Human Genome Project to designer babies; from the
war on cancer to Viagra; from the endless worry about prolonging life with
a healthy diet to the promise made by medical researchers that, although
death is inevitable, no particular disease is. Autonomy's greatest triumph
will come in the act of bringing human health, illness, and even death
into the realm of individual control and choice.

Medical care near the end of life provides an instructive example of
the process through which social policy and law have been deeply marked
by autonomy. When it comes to the use of life-sustaining medical
technology—ventilators, Intensive Care Units, dialysis, artificial nutrition

and hydration, cardio-pulmonary resuscitation, and the like—tailoring medical decisions to fit the individual's own values and preferences as closely as possible has had a salutatory effect. Such medical technology is often used very aggressively and thoughtlessly by highly specialized, technologically oriented and trained physicians. They are pressed for time and sometimes lose sight of the patient as a person in their zeal to use these powerful tools and medications to stave off death. These technologies rescue individuals from acute, possibly lethal, crises and prolong many lives, to be sure. However, in many cases their capacity to prolong biological functioning is not matched by a capacity to restore the patient to a meaningful quality of life or even conscious awareness and recognition of his surroundings or loved ones. These aggressive and invasive medical treatments and technologies serve only to prolong a person's dying, and may actively prolong suffering.

The law and medical ethics have found a way to allow the dying person to say no to additional futile treatment or to treatment that only prolongs the duration but not the quality of his life. This is one of the most important achievements in medicine since these powerful technologies began to be used and improved in the 1970s and 1980s. Appeals to the concept of autonomy have played a central role in the evolution of ethics and the law here. Still, the freedom of choice and decision purchased with the coin of autonomy is not without problems of its own. A kind of official, secular public philosophy of death and dying has been built around the individualistic and rationalistic assumptions of the concept of autonomy. That philosophy sits well with some dying persons and their families, but not with others. For some, autonomy at the end of life is a liberation; for others it turns out to be a substantial burden.[1]

Autonomy has clarified some of the ethical quandaries in end-of-life medical treatment, but it has done so at the cost of introducing a kind of formulaic, rule-oriented, and abstract mentality into medical care. This mentality can be blind to the real experiences and needs of dying persons and can be tone deaf to cultural and religious values and sensibilities that many people bring to their attempts to make sense of impending death or to grieve at impending loss. If we look back with a critical eye on the development of the ethical and legal framework of the right to die, we will find that a more relational and socially embedded understanding of the dying person can be appealed to in lieu of the excessively individualistic concept of autonomy. Doing so would grant families more trust and authority in cases where they must make end-of-life treatment decisions for loved ones who have lost the capacity to make decisions for themselves. It would give physicians something to appeal to when families make unreasonable and unwarranted demands for futile treatment that is not in the best interests—and does not serve the dignity—of the dying patient.

Above all, distinguishing between an ethic of end-of-life care governed by the notion of autonomy and such an ethic governed by the notion of preserving the patient's integrity as a person would provide a way of avoiding, as the logic of the concept of autonomy does not, the slippery slope of moving from legally recognizing the individual right to refuse life-sustaining medical treatment to the legalization of physician-assisted suicide (PAS) or active euthanasia.

The notion of autonomy in the face of death, or the so-called "right to die," has always been ambiguous. It has often been applied to the right to refuse medical treatment, but that is not really a right to die but rather a right to control what is done medically to your own body, the right to protect one's bodily integrity from invasive, unwanted, and unbeneficial medical treatment. The right to die is really an active right to aid or assistance in bringing about the end of one's life; it is a right to control, not one's medical care, but the precise timing and circumstances of one's death. Persons who refuse life-sustaining medical treatment often linger near death for a prolonged period of time, sometimes hours, sometimes days, sometimes even weeks. They may require strong pain medication and sedation to control their pain and suffering, and this medication may obscure their awareness or even put them into a kind of twilight sleep. Those who wish to assert the right to die in the strong sense, who want to exercise control over the circumstances of their dying, often reject this kind of lingering condition until biological systems shut down and natural death occurs. They want something quick, painless, effective, and neat.

This is the true ideal of last rights or self-sovereignty at the end of life. It is a logical extension of the ideal of a life lived on one's own terms, and only on those terms, throughout the course of adult life leading up to death. It is the fitting final chapter to the book of life as written by the culture of autonomy. It is also an exceedingly dangerous ideal and untenable as an ethical framework for end-of-life care. Legalizing physician-assisted suicide (as the state of Oregon has) or active medical euthanasia (as the

Netherlands has) is both an unnecessary and a dangerous policy proposal for the United States as a whole.

It is unnecessary because appropriate dignified care for the dying, through hospice and palliative care programs, for example, can be improved and made more widely available. These types of reforms would do more than legalizing PAS would to improve the admittedly inadequate care and support dying individuals often receive in the United States today.[2] It is no accident that hospice programs and professionals tend to oppose the legalization of PAS, for it is antithetical to their own philosophy, which is neither to hasten nor to prolong death. From their own clinical experience of caring for dying patients and their families hospice professionals also know that they can effectively treat the symptoms—pain, shortness of breath, enervation—and emotions—fear, loneliness, isolation, depression, dread—that ordinarily lead to suicidal wishes and impulses among the terminally ill.

It is dangerous because once medically assisted suicide or euthanasia became legally recognized, trust in the medical profession as a whole would likely erode. This is particularly true in an era of cost-containment when many patients already suspect that physicians are not necessarily acting in the patients' best interests. Regulation to prevent abuses would be difficult if not impossible, and subtle kinds of pressure and coercion—of a kind not at all justified by the conditions we have set forth in chapter 9— might be brought to bear on vulnerable individuals who would feel that accepting suicide rather than living with a terminal illness would be best for their family, would protect their finances, and would keep them from being a "burden" on others. Coercion in such instances is only one of the morally objectionable aspects. It is the culture of autonomy itself that largely is responsible for stigmatizing dependence and the need to rely on others. We put up with the dependency of children because we know they will grow out of it. But the dependency of the dying won't be left behind: it will last until the end. Our emphasis on autonomy as the condition that makes life worth living sends an overt message about how one should end one's life, even if tacitly the doctrine continues to include the freedom to choose even life-prolongation.

Is that the ethic of dying that we really ought to embrace, especially standing as we do on the brink of the aging society, the ending of the lives of tens of millions of Baby Boomers over the next three or four decades? We think not. Instead, society should be telling dying persons that their need and dependency is human and acceptable, not shameful. We should be telling them that it is acceptable for them to be a burden, for it is burden younger individuals, the healthy, and society as whole should welcome and gladly bear. We should be giving the dying among us more support for their final weeks and months, not a speedy exit.

In this chapter and the next we will explore the end-of-life care domain and the role of autonomy within it. In the remainder of this chapter we will examine the logic of autonomy in medical decisionmaking about the use of life-sustaining treatments and the limits and problems that the notion of autonomy leads to in that context. In the next chapter we will discuss the argument in favor of legalizing physician assisted suicide, particularly as that argument has appealed to autonomy as a moral and legal linchpin. Out of the debates in the end-of-life policy arena we seek to distill and fashion a notion of respect for the bodily integrity and social identity of the person. This notion, we believe, provides more adequate moral bearings in the difficult decisions that beset end-of-life care in hospitals, nursing homes, and ordinary homes throughout the country every day. And it also suggests a broader ethical vision of a life lived freely and responsibly in relationship and interdependency with others.

THE AMERICAN WAY OF DYING

In 1990 the U.S. Supreme Court held that the Constitution contains a "liberty interest" based in the Fourteenth Amendment, giving competent individuals the right to refuse all forms of life-sustaining medical treatment.[3] With this decision the so-called "right-to-die" movement gained an even more secure foothold in the public philosophy of America than it had enjoyed before, because the Constitution is the closest thing our secular, pluralistic society has to a common moral touchstone, a sacred text. Having established the right of the competent person to refuse treatment, the next question, which was the central issue before the court in the *Cruzan* case, is how this individual right to refuse treatment is to be exercised by others on behalf of persons lacking the capacity to decide for themselves. The role of family members and close friends in the twilight of the lives of the elderly, now and in the future, hangs in the balance.

Central to these and related questions are the notions of *rights* and *relationships*, notions that are profoundly shaped and defined by the framework and public philosophy now governing treatment decisionmaking at the end of life. In any public philosophy or framework there is a close interconnection among: (a) the way we define the rights of the self; (b) the way we think about the nature of the self; and (c) the way we evaluate interpersonal relationships, in other words, which relationships we publicly sanction and condone and which we consider illicit and threatening. Throughout this book we have argued that the ideas of rights, selfhood, and relationships as defined by the culture of autonomy are problematic in many ways. In applying autonomy to the ethics of medical care for the dying we encounter some blind spots that are particularly instructive. One noteworthy blind spot is the gap between the regulative ideals of the right to die or autonomy framework and the lived moral experience of the actual persons—physicians, family members, and patients—who make decisions near the end of life. This gap is a warning sign of something amiss in the moral imagination of the mainstream public philosophy itself. The quotidian moral experience of our familial and relational lives as selves—our social embeddedness as persons—may serve as a corrective to the aspiration for freedom or autonomy understood as moral self-sovereignty.

Shortly after the *Cruzan* decision Congress passed the Patient Self-Determination Act (PSDA),[4] which took effect in December 1991. Among other things, this law requires health care facilities to inform patients of their rights to execute an advance medical directive (i.e., a treatment directive commonly called a "living will" or a durable power of attorney for health care) and to document existing advance directives in the patient's medical records. The PSDA was a direct legislative response to the Supreme Court's *Cruzan* decision, which said that states may require rather strict procedural standards to ensure that physicians have "clear and convincing" evidence of the patient's wishes before life-sustaining treatment can be terminated at the request of a family member or other surrogate.

Advance directives executed by the still competent patient are thought to satisfy all the necessary procedural requirements, and hence contain the practical key to the individual's theoretical moral and legal right to refuse treatment. By the end of the 1990s virtually every state in the union had either a statute or a court ruling recognizing the validity and the importance of advance directives as a means of keeping the patient's own voice at the center of end-of-life decisionmaking. The problem is that fewer than 20 percent of people nationwide are believed to have completed such an advance directive, and critically ill patients regularly show up at hospitals or reside in nursing homes for whom there is no clear record of what the patient would have wanted. In these cases family members, if there are any present, or close friends must serve as "surrogate decisionmakers."

Visiting a senior center in the early 1990s, Bruce Jennings, one of the authors, once heard an elderly African American gentleman express an attitude that is at odds with the autonomy framework but is nonetheless apparently rather widespread. This outspoken gentleman, although he seemed to understand quite well what advance directives were, would have no truck with them. "I reckon my family is my advance directive," he said.

The conventional wisdom of the right to die framework would say that this gentleman is making a big mistake. His attitude, although perhaps touching and charming, is dangerously out of step with our current public policy. His attitude is dangerous to him, and to his family, because it puts him and them at risk of being effectively disenfranchised should he lose decisionmaking capacity. What would they do if he ever gets to the point where they know, but cannot prove clearly, that he would say, enough is enough?

It is not difficult to describe briefly how this man's statement is out of step with current public policy, and we will turn to that in a moment. Even more important, though, is to see philosophically *why* his attitude is out of step, why the very notion that one's family can be one's advance directive is incoherent from the point of view of the autonomy framework.

The reason is that to find his statement meaningful and coherent you have to have a different conception of the self from autonomy's conception, and a different conception of the intimate relationships that, at the best of times, characterize connections between family members and close friends. It is necessary to see the self, not as a subject that is *in* relationships, but as the subject *of* relationships—a dynamic process of identity in which the self both constitutes its relationships to others and is constituted by them. And it is necessary to see the "family" as a community of intimate connectedness, rather than the way it is often portrayed (although no one these days would dare try to define it): a functional economic or reproductive unit, or a grouping of genetically related individuals held together, if at all, by a habit of propinquity, deep-seated sentiments of affection and familiarity, or mutual advantage.

The relational self and the family as a community of intimate connectedness—autonomy accommodates neither of these views readily, if at all. Our mainstream public philosophy of dying is based on the notion that there should be no socially imposed conception of euthanasia—good death or good dying. In a 1983 report that has become almost the *locus classicus* of the right-to-die framework, the President's Commission on Ethical Problems in Medicine formulated this notion in the following terms: "The Commission argued that decisions about the treatments that best promote a patient's health and well-being must be based on the particular patient's values and goals; no uniform, objective determination can be adequate—whether defined by society or by health professionals. . . . [T]he primacy of a patient's interests in self-determination and in honoring the patient's own view of well-being warrant leaving with the patient the final authority to decide."[5]

This view is consonant with the position in recent political theory that has come to be known as the thesis of liberal neutrality. According to this theory, individuals should enjoy self-sovereignty over the meaning of aspects of the good life, including good dying, as the good pertains primarily or exclusively to them alone.

In other words, the dramatic question, "Whose life is it, anyway?" could just as well have been "Whose death is it, anyway?" The answer would have been the same: mine. Not ours. John Donne's marvelous trope is turned upside down.[6] The funeral bell does not toll for the entire community, and our mortality is not, as Donne would have it, a fundamentally equalizing and binding force of shared vulnerability, frailty, and dependency. In contemporary America the bell tolls eventually for each of us, to be sure, but it tolls for us one at a time.

The cardinal sin, then, is to impose an alien conception of the good onto the nonconsenting self, thereby abridging self-sovereignty in the definition of good dying. That alien conception can come from society as a whole (usually represented by the state), or from any other person—stranger or friend, relative or not, intimate or mere associate, it doesn't matter for the purposes of protecting this special and fundamental sort of liberty. So long as others are not harmed, and their rights are not violated, all persons should be allowed to follow their own conception of the good: to live their life in their own way, and to die their death in their own way.

The Right-to-Die Framework and Its Problems

Once we grasp the pivotal role played by the aspiration to achieve and to protect self-sovereignty over the definition of one's good, the particular form taken by most ethical and legal arguments concerning decisions to forgo life-sustaining treatment makes perfect sense.

Start with the right (liberty) of the competent patient to refuse treatment, without paternalistic interference from physicians or anybody else. Then move to the harder cases of surrogate decisionmaking, when family members are usually involved as the surrogate. The adversarial posture assumed by discussions of the right of the competent patient does not lessen; if anything, it intensifies. The right to refuse treatment survives the loss of capacity. The sovereign moral will of the patient must still be empowered and protected; that will must be given voice by indirect means. The goal then is to make the surrogate the selfless instrument of the patient's sovereign will. The danger is that the surrogate has his own will, his own self, his own fears, values, beliefs, and conceptions of good living and good dying. An order of surrogate decision rules has emerged that is designed to promote that goal and avert that danger. Lurking behind these rules is the specter of the surrogate as adversary—an alien will, an other self, vying to control the decisionmaking power at the expense of the easily forgotten, vulnerable will or voice of the patient.

The rules are as follows.[7] First, follow the instructions of the patient's treatment directive, if there is one and if it reasonably pertains to the clinical situation of the patient. Second, follow the counterfactual thought experiment called "substituted judgment." Based on an inference about what is generally known about the patient's values and beliefs, and from the way the patient lived his or her life, the surrogate should try to reconstruct the decision that the patient would make if the patient could decide. Note that this decision rule is also patient-centered: it is the patient's beliefs and wishes that count, not the surrogate's. Finally, if there is no advance directive and if not enough is known about the patient to make a reasonable inference, then the surrogate should do what is in the "best interests" of the patient. Here best interests are not to be defined as the surrogate himself or herself would define them, but as a hypothetical "reasonable person" would. Again, the purpose of this exercise in hypothetical reasoning is to keep the dangerous subjectivity of the surrogate as far removed from the moral and epistemological basis of the treatment decision as possible.

This framework has been subjected to constant and largely critical scrutiny for many years.[8] Much of the discussion has focused on the substituted judgment and the best interest standards. It is apparent that these are rather strict and demanding standards when stated in the abstract and enunciated by the courts. Unable to draw such rigid lines between their own will and that of a loved one, real life surrogates and family members regularly fail to live up to these standards in practice. On those relatively rare occasions when termination of treatment cases do go to court, judges regularly accept practical decisions made by family members, but then must go to considerable—sometimes implausible—lengths to show that the incompetent patient, not the family, "really" made the decision. Most courts recognize that out of practical necessity they must trust and empower families, and in effect they do so, but only when family power can be made legally invisible.

Why the inconsistency? One reason is because abandoning the strict formal standards would too clearly countenance the fact that terminal care decisionmaking as it is actually practiced is empowering something other than the sovereign self and will of the patient, considered as an isolated and separate individual. To admit this is a scandal in the culture of autonomy. To avoid this agonal clash of competing wills in a struggle over what will be done to the body of the patient requires a different understanding of who the patient is, and a different understanding of the moral authority that flows to the surrogate by dint of a certain type of (past and present) relationship with the patient. But these altered understandings remain unavailable to the right to die framework as it is presently constituted.

At the moment the framework of last rights is evolving in two dimensions. On the one hand, it is apparent that the best course is to fall back on the presence of an advance directive. Surrogates guided by them are on the firmest moral ground. On the other hand, no matter how much effort is put into public education and encouraging people to make out advance directives, a substantial number of incompetent patients will remain without one. To cope with this reality, a recent trend has been the passage of state laws that explicitly authorize family members, usually in some stipulated order of preference, to make treatment decisions.

It is not yet clear how future statutes of this type will be written or how those that pass will be interpreted. Perhaps these laws may portend a movement away from the current framework of surrogate decisionmaking and toward a more open-ended recognition of the rights of family members as such to make these decisions. On the other hand, some proposed laws and recent court rulings, such as the *Martin* case in Michigan[9] and the *Wendland* case in California,[10] place some onerous procedural obstacles in the path of family members who opt to forgo life-sustaining treatments. Trust is the scarcest resource in the American health care system today.

Where can we go from here? In the last few years public policy regarding decisions near the end of life has been abuzz with activity, with new statutes, regulations, and guidelines being promulgated each year. This activity is misleading, however, because it masks an underlying stasis or paralysis in our thinking. Our legislators and policy makers are like builders constructing an addition to a house, but making up the plan as they go along. They have no overall design in mind, no sense of proportion or of what shape the overall structure should be. Without that design, they have no idea when to stop building. How much law is enough in the area of terminal care?

It is a misleading metaphor to think of ethics as a detailed blueprint for public policy. However, if our diagnosis is correct, end-of-life care policy is aimless because some of the fundamental philosophical conceptions underlying it are in disarray. The official stories we tell ourselves about what we are supposed to be doing are out of sync with much of the lived reality of terminal care. As we have seen, the current policy consensus is centered on the right of the individual patient to refuse any and all forms of medical treatment, including life-sustaining treatment. It is an individualistic and autonomy-respecting consensus. Because it places such emphasis on the voice of the patient in the decisionmaking process, one of its main goals is to continue to be guided by that voice as much as possible, even when the patient has lost decisionmaking capacity and can no longer speak or decide for himself. Hence the emphasis that has been placed on educating patients to fill out advance directives.

Unfortunately this consensus alone will not be enough in the twenty-first century. Already some ragged edges are appearing in the end-of-life care consensus, and these may lead us to reconsider its underlying philosophy as well as its practical implementation.

The excessive rationalism of the consensus. The consensus works best for those who plan ahead for their terminal illness. Most Americans find that exceedingly hard to do. The denial of death and the reluctance of individuals to engage in advance planning remain very strong in mainstream American culture. The number of people who prepare advance directives remains abysmally small. The consensus forces us to acknowledge the limits of what medicine can promise and the limits of our own mortality.

The excessive individualism of the consensus. Patient autonomy is the cornerstone, ethically and sociologically, of the way we have approached decisions near the end of life since the early 1970s. The legacy of that emphasis has produced a movement in favor not just of the right to refuse medical treatment, but also the right to medical assistance with suicide. The end of life is not the best time to wage battles on behalf of autonomy. Caring, family, mutual respect and love, and attentiveness to the dying person are the qualities most needed then. Our consensus has if anything been rather distrusting of families, and tends to make them morally invisible in the official dying process. They are empty conduits of the patient's wishes. Mothers and fathers, brothers and sisters, relatives lose their names in bioethics and become "surrogates" or "proxies," appropriately cold terms to denote an impersonal role.

The middle-class cultural bias of the consensus. Already suggested by the rationalism and the individualism of the consensus, this framework for decisionmaking at the end of life does not travel well across cultures and traditions within our increasingly pluralistic society. Durable powers of attorney for health care may be translated into many languages, but substantively they may often be incomprehensible. Is planning and decisionmaking the only or the most appropriate response to the recognition that one is dying? Is everyone's first thought a concern to protect the family from being burdened? How does one respond to the suspicion, built up over a lifetime of experiencing discrimination, that advance directives are racist documents designed to limit resources offered to persons of color?

The misdiagnosis of the problem. The consensus has always believed that inappropriately aggressive and unwanted treatment at the end of life is fundamentally a problem of prognostic uncertainty and poor communication. And yet, as the SUPPORT study demonstrated, physician behavior is not altered significantly by addressing uncertainty and poor communication alone. These are elements of the physician-patient relationship seen as a personal interaction. The fundamental problem with end-of-life care, however, may be structural and institutional in nature. In the modern acute care hospital virtually everything is oriented toward the use of life-sustaining equipment and techniques, not to forgoing them. The informal culture of specialty medicine, the reward system, the institutional pressures faced by family members, the range of choices people *in extremis* are being asked to make—each of these factors and more are part of a system that is extremely resistant to change when confronted with an ideal, counter-cultural decisionmaking model, even one that is supported by the force of law and professional ethics.

The solution to these problems is not yet clear. Perhaps a countervailing system—one oriented toward palliative and hospice care—needs to be created to give at least one real alternative to patients and families. It is hard to see how anything short of this alternative system (which exists now in bits and pieces but serves only about one in five dying persons) will suffice. Until then we will continue to urge individuals to prepare for death in advance, and we will continue to require them to make a series of agonizing micro-decisions in order to stay on the right pathway toward death.

A DEATH IN THE FAMILY

Let us return to the second unresolved problem with the right-to-die framework, its excessive individualism, and consider the role of the family more deeply. The role, rights, and responsibilities of the family is an issue no less contentious in the realm of end-of-life care than it is in other areas of social policy. The recent literature on family roles and rights in termination of treatment decisions contains some interesting attempts to carve out a broader moral justification for family decision makers without fundamentally departing from the right to die framework. Nancy Rhoden, for example, offers a procedural solution by legally shifting the burden of proof from the family member, who now often must show that his or her decision is what the patient would have wanted. Rhoden would have the courts place the burden of proof on anyone who challenges the family's decision to show that the decision is not reasonable and cannot reasonably be construed as consonant with the patient's values or interests. She also softens the adversarial image of patient/family relationships so common in the bioethics and legal literature, arguing that it is empirically overstated and cannot be the guiding assumption of public policy and the law.[11]

A different theoretical tack is taken by ethicist John Hardwig, who embraces an adversarial view of patient/family relationships, but argues on grounds of justice that distinct family interests are at stake and should be taken into account in end-of-life decisions.[12] His strategy, in effect, is to move the right to die from the domain of the good into the domain of the right, where liberal theory has ample conceptual resources and historical experience as a public philosophy for dealing with distributive justice and conflicting rights claims. For Hardwig decisions about end-of-life care become a question of fairly distributing the benefits and burdens of the decision between the dying person and other members of the family, especially those whose lives and plans will be disrupted by the burdens of caregiving should the patient's life with severe dependency and disability be prolonged by medical means. Moreover, there is no reason, in this view, to stop at the boundaries of the family unit: the interests of society as a whole, or a large group of premium payers in an insurance pool, might equally be pitted against the individual interests of the patient in this contest for fair and just distribution. For others are others, and there is no moral or sociological differentiation between other individuals who are related by kinship and marriage and others who are related to the self by different types of social ties, including very abstract, impersonal, and economic ones. The type of analysis differentiating family from state, market, and civil society that we sketched in chapter 9 is missing from this analysis of distributive justice in an essentially undifferentiated social group.

Moving further away from the view of the unencumbered self and the purely instrumental value of interpersonal relationships, James L. Nelson argues that a special class of durable and intimate relationships should be perceived as having intrinsic moral value.[13] These bonds, where individuals do not necessarily define themselves as separate from the relationship, should be respected by public policies and procedures in all aspects of health care. Social arrangements that have the effect of imposing separateness and division where the individuals involved may rather see connections and commonality of interest are no less objectionable than the paternalistic impositions that autonomy and the right to die framework has been so concerned to avoid.

We concur with Nelson's approach, but would push these notions further and in yet another direction. Nelson's argument still sets the self's relationships in opposition to separate—and presumably nonrelational— aspects of the self's own interests. This allows him to strengthen the hand of the self's commitment to relationships relative to the self's other interests. However, instead of bolstering relationships by granting them a more substantial kind of value, perhaps we need to rethink the assumptions about the self that allow it to have interests apart from relationships in the first place.

Families matter. When the elderly African American gentleman at the senior center called his family his advance directive, he was locating his family within the horizon of value that made his own life matter. And he was singling his family out, giving it pride of place. He was saying that he didn't live merely with or in his family, but through them, and they through him. He was saying that somehow who those family members were, and the community of connectedness and commitment his family was, expressed his identity—his self. His family members did not merely transmit his will, his voice, like the wires of a telephone. They also embodied his will, they gave it shape and life. At some point they were all of his will there was left.

The framework of last rights is best understood, we believe, as a localized instance of what we have been calling the culture of autonomy or what Charles Taylor has called "the culture of authenticity." The general strategy Taylor recommends is not to reject the development of modern individualism root and branch, as if we could return to some premodern sense of community, nor to transcend it altogether in some postmodern deconstruction of the self. Instead we should attempt an internal critique of this aspiration to self-sovereignty. Such a critique would, in effect, attempt to rescue autonomy from itself; it would try to show that what is truly liberating and humanely affirming in this framework is not itself well served or adequately expressed in the concrete forms of argument, social practice, and public policy that have been justified in its name.[14] We agree.

One essential part of this task is to recognize that contemporary liberalism, with its ideals of individualism and autonomy, is itself a theory of the human good. At times and in the hands of some authors, it is a robust vision of human flourishing that is by no means indefensible. Many leading liberal theorists, such as John Rawls and Ronald Dworkin, deny this.[15]

Another central point to be developed has to do with the necessarily social and contextual character of all human language, meaning, and conceptions such as the good itself. From this perspective the notion that an individual can unilaterally define his or her own good is incoherent. It is based on a vision of moral will and choice abstracted from all contexts or horizons of value located beyond or outside the self. However, this abstraction deprives both will and choice of any point because it strips away everything that could make will and choice matter. Human freedom has three faces, not just two: *freedom from* oppression, *freedom to* flourish, and *freedom for* something that matters. A horizonless choice is an empty choice; freedom exercised for its own sake, pointing to nothing beyond itself, creates a hollow self.

This chapter began with references to two very different texts, the *Book of Common Prayer* and the Supreme Court's *Cruzan* decision. Each reminds us of a moral ideal: the blessings of care, on one side, and self-determination or self-sovereignty, on the other. We cannot abandon either of these ideals. We must recover them and make them live afresh in a way that makes them complimentary rather than conflicting. Unless we do this we shall grow old alone.

When our deepest experience at crucial transitions in life is at odds with the public vocabularies of value and meaning available to us, we have a crisis of thought and spirit too unsettling to ignore. We need to return to the roots of this crisis and remember that liberalism and the vindication of human rights was once a call for equal personal dignity and mutual respect in a community of shared purpose. Concepts such as autonomy, the right to die, self-sovereignty and self-determination are only one vocabulary, and a bare one at that, with which to advance this notion of human self-realization.

It is not necessary to confront imminent death to understand the importance of a sense of self that goes beyond one's own skin. Many of us, young and old, understand it well enough in our everyday experience of family. Others have families that are stony ground, but they still may cultivate this sensibility in other places. But our public language and our moral ideal of autonomy fails to acknowledge and to nourish that understanding.

12

Last Rights II: Autonomy, Moral Trespass, and Physician-Assisted Suicide

> [The human being] is a person who within the ambience of the flesh claims our care.... He is therefore a sacredness in illness and in his dying.... The sanctity of human life prevents ultimate trespass upon him even for the sake of treating his bodily life....
>
> —PAUL RAMSEY, *The Patient as Person*

MEDICAL TREATMENT NEAR the end of life and the care of the dying are among the most important issues facing medicine in the aging society. How imaginatively will moral and legal discourse respond to the fundamental human challenge of accepting our mortality? The answer to this question will determine, in large measure, how well or badly most of us alive today shall die.

A version of philosophical and political liberalism—"liberal neutrality"—holds the key to how well society will respond to this challenge. The theory of liberal neutrality holds that public power should not be used to favor any particular conception of the human good, but must remain impartial among competing conceptions.[1] This neutral liberalism, which purports to leave all questions of the human good up to the personal choice of individuals is, of course, the flip side of the culture of autonomy. Neutral liberalism, attractive as it is in many ways, is ultimately a neutered liberalism. It provides an unduly abstract and individualistic public philosophy of death and dying. It puts more ethical weight on individual rights to personal control than these rights will bear, and it fails to refine the concepts of reciprocity, mutuality, and

229

interdependency. These are precisely the concepts that are essential to the moral language of a genuinely multigenerational society of caregiving and common respect.

Liberal neutrality has three basic tenets: first, the doctrine of the moral primacy of the right over the good; second, the legal primacy of individual rights over collective considerations of social utility; and third, the political primacy of noninterference, impartiality, and neutrality on the part of the state in relation to beliefs held by individuals and groups, such as religious communities, about the nature of the human good and the good life. The first of these is generally in keeping with a deontological meta-ethic, drawn from the contractarian tradition in ethics and political theory. The other two tenets are consistent with the type of constitutional liberalism that has developed in the United States, particularly in the postwar period and the modern civil rights era.

According to this version of liberalism, matters promoting a measure of egalitarian social justice and protecting individual rights are properly the concern of the democratic state, whereas matters of more positive duty concerning human self-realization and the good are matters of private belief. About such private beliefs a liberal society as a whole will never agree, and the state must take a neutral role, enforcing only meta-norms of tolerance and mutual respect.

The theory of liberal neutrality is the policy arm of the right-to-die debate. As we discussed in chapter 11, this debate began as an attempt to empower patients, or their surrogates, in decisionmaking about the use of life-sustaining medical technologies. That argument has run its course from the 1976 New Jersey State Supreme Court decision in *In re Quinlan*[2] to the 1990 U.S. Supreme Court's *Cruzan* decision. By the early 1990s, the patient's right to refuse treatment, even life-sustaining treatment, was legally and morally secure for the most part, though it was far from being fully respected in actual medical practice. But the battle over the legalization of physician-assisted suicide (PAS) was beginning, and the right-to-die debate in America opened a new chapter.

Is there any moral and legal difference between the right to forgo unwanted but life-prolonging medical treatment, on the one hand, and the right to determine the precise nature, circumstances, and timing of one's own death, on the other?

THE DECADE OF DEATH AND DYING

The 1990s will be remembered as a decade marked by an increasing social awareness of death and dying. The decade began with the United States Supreme Court's first landmark ruling on end-of-life care in *Cruzan*, in which the Court recognized that a right to refuse life-sustaining treatment may exist. In *Cruzan*, the Court found that under certain circumstances a surrogate may act for the patient in determining end-of-life decisions. Following this decision, a number of different approaches addressing end-of-life care arose. Congress passed the Patient Self-Determination Act, and durable powers of attorney for health care statutes appeared in many states, along with public education efforts to encourage the use of advance directives. These approaches all focused on the importance of considering individual preference about end-of-life care.

Approximately two million foreseeable deaths occur each year in the United States, more than half of those take place in a hospital or other health care facility, and in those institutions as many as 70 percent of the deaths come after some deliberate nontreatment decision (including a do-not-resuscitate order) has been made.

In the mid-1990s, the SUPPORT study provided rigorous documentation of the alarming extent to which aggressive life-prolonging measures were still being used in situations where they were either medically futile or were unwanted by the patients, or both.[3] Even concerted efforts to improve communication between physicians and dying patients did not stem the technological momentum of end-of-life care in the country's major medical centers. Moreover, a large proportion of families reported postmortem that the patient had spent the last two or three days of life in severe, unrelieved pain.

Growing public fears of losing control of care at the end of life—of becoming dependent on machines, of being an emotional and financial burden to one's family, and of suffering due to inadequate treatment of pain and other symptoms—led to a remarkable grassroots movement in the late 1990s to legalize physician-assisted suicide. The fears of an aging society were dramatized by the public defiance of Dr. Jack Kevorkian, the debate over the Oregon referendum that legalized PAS for the first time in the United States, and by the Federal Appeals Court rulings in the Second and Ninth Circuits, *Quill v. Vacco*[4] and *Compassion in Dying v.*

Washington[5] that temporarily struck down existing state laws against PAS before those appellate rulings were overturned by the U.S. Supreme Court in the summer of 1997 (*Vacco v. Quill* and *Washington v. Glucksberg*). However, the Supreme Court refused to interfere with the Oregon law,[6] and it left the constitutional door open to other states to change their laws on PAS as they saw fit.

Since that time a referendum to legalize PAS has failed to pass in Michigan, and another has failed in Maine. Dr. Kevorkian has been convicted of murder and sentenced to prison for ending the life of a man with advanced ALS (amyotrophic lateral sclerosis, more commonly known as "Lou Gehrig's Disease").

Clearly we cannot suppress the question of what counts as a good death. In spite of all the remarkable attention and energy that has been devoted to wrestling with that notion in the 1990s, a firm grasp on it continues to elude us because it has thus far been addressed as what the sociologist C. Wright Mills once called "a personal trouble," rather than as a "civic problem."[7] A personal trouble resides within the individual's own heart and mind. A civic problem, by contrast, reveals the connection between what individuals experience in their personal and family lives and the larger structures of society that surround them.

Dying, that most intimate and private of personal experiences, is not *only* a personal experience; what dying involves is socially and culturally shaped. In order to address the question of a good dying as a civic question— that is, one that engages the shared values of a community of diverse faiths, backgrounds, and needs—it is necessary to confront prevailing arguments that render such questions suspect or illegitimate in principle. That is precisely why the paradigm of liberal neutrality must be challenged.

APPLYING LIBERAL NEUTRALITY TO PHYSICIAN-ASSISTED SUICIDE

Liberal neutrality structures the moral imagination in particular ways so that certain questions come to the foreground whereas others recede. It finds its most intelligent and uncompromising application to bioethics in the work of philosopher and legal theorist Ronald Dworkin.

In *Life's Dominion*, Dworkin wants to show that the culture wars over both abortion and "euthanasia" can be resolved by recourse to the tenets of liberal neutrality theory.[8] The sanctity of life and the value one places on prolonged life under different states of impairment and quality of life are fundamental components of a conception of the human good, Dworkin observes. Reasonable persons in an open society will disagree about the sanctity of life. The role of law and public morality is to preserve the space of that disagreement and of plural ways of living in accordance with one's beliefs.[9] It is not the role of law to settle such disagreements nor to bring the coercive power of the state down on one side or another in this dispute.[10]

If we cannot reasonably agree on when life begins or on the relative value of fetal life, Dworkin contends, and if we cannot reasonably agree on when dying begins or on the relative value of living while dying, then in both cases the law should not be used to interfere with the individual's liberty to act on the basis of her considered beliefs. This liberty of conscience makes policy questions concerning abortion and euthanasia analogous to constitutional questions about religious freedom. Moreover, the individual's interest in controlling the circumstances of the disposition of his or her own body and fundamental life activities, which Dworkin dubs "critical interests," make these issues akin to constitutional issues of liberty under the Fourteenth Amendment.

This line of reasoning leads Dworkin to the conclusion that the Supreme Court was correct, although not always for the right reasons, in the abortion cases. The state should not interfere with a woman's freedom to continue or to discontinue her pregnancy because to do so is to impose one group's conception of the good coercively onto nonconsenting individuals who do not share those private beliefs.

The same reasoning applies, *mutatis mutandis*, to laws pertaining to the refusal of life-sustaining medical treatment, physician-assisted suicide, and even voluntary active euthanasia. The case law from *Quinlan* to *Cruzan* was correct to affirm the right of the individual to refuse life-sustaining medical treatment, Dworkin argues, because to use the power of the state to force unwanted treatment onto patients would be to give official sanction to some private conceptions of the sanctity of life. Finally, because there is no principled difference between the refusal of life-sustaining treatment and requesting assistance with dying via lethal prescription (PAS) or lethal injection (active euthanasia), statutes making it a crime for physicians to aid in dying should be overturned as unconstitutional. Doing so would affirm, once again, that the substantive political morality enshrined in the Constitution is essentially that of liberal neutrality.

Dworkin and several other distinguished American moral philosophers (Thomas Nagel, Robert Nozick, John Rawls, Thomas Scanlon, and Judith Jarvis Thomson) entered the controversy over the legalization of physician-assisted suicide when they prepared an *amicus curiae* (friend of the court) brief supporting the prolegalization side and submitted it to the U.S. Supreme Court. This document became known as the "Philosophers' Brief." It is essentially a statement of the liberal neutrality perspective applied to the question of legalizing PAS. It follows closely the version of that theory put forward in *Life's Dominion*.

If affirmed by the Supreme Court, the PAS cases would have replayed a scenario like that created by *Roe v. Wade*.[11] With the finding of a constitutionally protected right for individuals, the court would have swept aside existing statutes in nearly every state, creating the need for a long series of other rulings to fine tune what statutory approaches were permissible. This is precisely what liberally neutral courts are supposed to do in a democracy. On the other hand, such an exercise of judicial power might have triggered a bitter social conflict akin to that which has persisted around abortion since *Roe v. Wade*. Few issues have been better positioned recently to illustrate the principles of liberal neutrality.

In an introduction to the brief added when it was reprinted in the *New York Review of Books*, Dworkin left no doubt about the continuity between the brief and the theory of liberal neutrality: "The Philosophers' Brief," he writes, "defines a very general moral and constitutional principle that every competent person has the right to make momentous personal decisions which invoke fundamental religious or philosophical convictions about life's value for himself."[12] The brief itself asserts that denying competent, terminally ill patients, who find their continued life intolerable, the freedom to hasten their own death, or to ask others for help in doing so, is something improper for the state to do. This is due to the fact that "individuals have a constitutionally protected interest in making those grave judgments for themselves, free from the imposition of any religious or philosophical orthodoxy by court or legislature." For the state to deny such persons the "opportunity" to hasten their death "could only be justified on the basis of a religious or ethical conviction about the value or meaning of life itself. Our Constitution forbids government to impose such convictions on its citizens."[13]

The body of the brief then goes on to consider other potential justifications for denying this liberty and finds them all wanting. It also argues that prior court rulings in other areas of medical care decisionmaking, reproductive decisions, and privacy establish the basis for the proposition that there is a constitutionally protected liberty interest to allow individuals to make momentous life choices free from the imposition of any religious or philosophical orthodoxy. Finally, it contends that to decide to hasten one's death, for any personal reason, is one of those constitutionally protected areas of our liberty.

Both *Life's Dominion* and the "Philosophers' Brief" share a common problem: how to persuade anyone not already predisposed to agree to accept the basic starting point of the entire argument. That premise is the notion that state prohibition on ending the life of one's fetus with medical assistance or ending one's own life with medical assistance is properly understood as a violation of a fundamental individual right and an unconstitutional imposition of a religious or philosophical orthodoxy on citizens. A more straightforward view of the matter is that a valid purpose of the state is to prevent one person from directly and intentionally killing another, and that is what laws against abortion and PAS are all about.

One may argue that this legitimate state purpose is misdirected in the case of particular laws against abortion or PAS, or that other rights or social interests outweigh this state interest in discouraging intentional killing. But those are not the arguments that Dworkin or the theory of liberal neutrality generally pursue, and they would not constitute the radical paradigm shift in our moral understanding of individual rights that Dworkin hopes to accomplish. Why should one take freedom of conscience rather than intentional killing to be the central issue raised by PAS? He does not supply independent reasons for why one should do so.

Another troubling aspect of Dworkin's argument that many may find objectionable is that he tends to transform ideas that many people regard as objective moral truth into matters of irrational belief. In a word, he transforms a good deal of the content of what some people regard as public morality into the realm of private religion, and he seems to do this sorting in an arbitrary or ideologically motivated way.

Drawing the line between public morals and private religion is crucial in a liberal society, but Dworkin again does not provide much in the way of justification for doing so. This is all the more troubling because he focuses so much of his work on the policymaking role of judges and the courts, and seems to give little place for democratic politics or representational policymakers in the realm of social policy that touches on fundamental individual rights. This is a shortcoming of the theory of liberal neutrality generally: it relies far too heavily on effecting progressive social change through judicial authority and betrays an orientation toward politics generally that is elitist and antidemocratic.

Concerning the argument of the "Philosophers' Brief" itself, some of our concerns are as follows. First, do past court decisions in the abortion and termination of treatment cases actually require finding a constitutionally protected right to assistance in controlling the timing of one's death? Second, even though the cases under review were about provisions in state law that penalize physicians if they assist in suicide, the argument actually put forward by the brief gives grounds for saying that an individual has a right to obtain the assistance of anyone he chooses (and who agrees), not only a physician. It is actually an argument for assisted suicide, not physician-assisted suicide.

Moreover, it is not merely an argument for assisted suicide but also one for direct euthanasia. There is no reason given why the dying patient must take her life with her own hand. Doctors may write a prescription for pills the patient takes, or loved ones may hand her a gun; doctors may also administer an injection, and loved ones may pull the trigger. Our emotional or aesthetic responses to any of these scenarios do not factor into the analysis at all. Interestingly, however, sympathy for the plight of the dying, especially the moving cases represented by the plaintiffs in the cases, does figure in the brief, but not directly in its conceptual or argumentative structure. These considerations are clearly intended to move the reader as rhetorical ornamentation.

Finally, the "Philosophers' Brief" asserts that no other justification can be given for prohibiting PAS other than the unacceptable imposition of some kind of metaphysical orthodoxy on the citizens of a pluralistic society. *Amicus* briefs are necessarily compact and terse. With such severe space limitations, it was a dubious decision on the part of the authors to devote so much discussion to the straw man notion of the distinction between acts and omissions. What they needed to address, and what the majority opinion by Justice Rehnquist ultimately relied on and embraced, was the distinction between the right to be free of unwanted bodily invasion versus the right to obtain assistance in directly and deliberately ending one's life. Using rhetoric and phraseology that erases that important distinction, the "Philosophers' Brief" does not take it seriously nor address it adequately.

A Critique of Liberal Neutrality

We turn now to the more general implications and effects of the liberal neutrality framework. Viewing the right-to-die issue through the lens of liberal neutrality affects our understanding in several important respects. First, it links a localized question—"How should we regulate medical practice and the use of medical technology in given areas of practice?"— with a societal issue about the nature of our constitutional regime. To restrict abortion would not simply restrict the freedom of women (or protect the unborn), it would threaten civil and religious liberties across the board. Liberal neutrality would have us come to believe the same thing about laws governing both the termination of life-sustaining treatment, PAS, and active euthanasia.

Second, this perspective sets up a linear narrative for the development of the right-to-die debate. According to this narrative, individual autonomy at the end of life is a logical extension of the entire civil rights movement of the postwar years. These questions do not arise primarily because people are living longer, nor because advances of medical technology prolong biological life beyond the capacity to restore function or cognitive capacity and may be prolonging the process of dying in a burdensome way. These questions arise for an altogether different reason: they represent the next frontier in sweeping away the legal residue of a past era when individuals were subject to foreign or outside conceptions of the good and conceptions of how they should live their lives (or die their deaths) without any sufficient public warrant (such as protecting others against harm or violation of their rights).

The liberal neutrality perspective erases the distinction between the right to refuse life-sustaining treatment and the right to obtain medical assistance with one's death from a physician. It offers no moral grounds for such a distinction, whereas that distinction has emerged as a linchpin of bioethics and the law when only forgoing life-supports was the center of attention.

This is important for the sake of ethical and jurisprudential consistency. If there is no principled distinction to be made between forgoing treatment and PAS, and if the courts have decided against a prohibition on the practice of forgoing treatment, then the courts cannot consistently allow a prohibition on the practice of PAS either. If there is a common law right or liberty interest at work, it is the person's right to choose death or control the timing and circumstances of one's own death. In both forgoing treatment and PAS the patient exercises the same right, not two different rights, and the patient and the physician have the same goal, namely, the early death of the patient and the relief of suffering caused by pro-longed living.

The question is also important for a constitutional reason. If there is no principled distinction to be made between the two, and the courts permit decisions to forgo life-sustaining treatment but prohibit PAS, then this state of affairs may itself be in violation of the equal protection clause of the Fourteenth Amendment. The law may ban both, or permit both, but it cannot split the difference. This in essence is what the Federal Appeals Court for the Second Circuit held in *Quill v. Vacco*.

Finally, it is important politically, both within the Supreme Court and in the broader political arena. Within the court, it is important for the sake of the rule of *stare decisis*. Many of those who argued in favor of PAS in the Supreme Court cases of 1997, *Washington v. Glucksberg* and *Vacco v. Quill*, warned the court that if it upheld the existing prohibition in state laws against PAS, then the ruling would undermine important earlier precedents in both the abortion and the right-to-refuse-treatment areas. In particular, a ruling against PAS could not be reconciled with either *Planned Parenthood v. Casey*[14] or with *Cruzan*. The prospect of this legal implication put those who support abortion rights but are hesitant about the right to PAS in an awkward and uncomfortable position.

For the liberal neutrality perspective to deny the moral force of the distinction between forgoing treatment and PAS or active euthanasia is also ironic. In the late 1970s and early 1980s, vitalists and others associated with the right to life movement opposed decisions to forgo life-sustaining treatment on two grounds. The first was that this was no different from murder. The second was the argument that once high tech medical treat-ment could be forgone, then there would be no way to stem the movement toward forgoing medically provided nutrition and hydration, then toward giving high doses of narcotics, and finally to intentional killing of the patient.

After two decades, forgoing treatment has gained legal, ethical, and medical legitimacy, and the right-to-die movement has turned its attention to active, intentional medically assisted dying (as have the right to life and the disability rights movements in opposition). This time what was previously anathema is now seeking acceptance and justification. Openly advocating that physicians may intend the death of a patient works to elevate PAS rather than to cast a pall over forgoing treatment. In the American right-to-die debate we have come full circle.

CAREFUL LANGUAGE AT THE END OF LIFE

As an ethical and legal consensus emerged from 1976 to 1990, the distinction between forgoing treatment and suicide or assisting suicide became fundamental. In the right-to-die cases, the burden of proof lies with the state or with those who would impose restrictions on individual liberty. Is there a proportionally compelling state or societal interest at stake that justifies the restriction of liberty? And are the least restrictive means being used to achieve this important social end?

In conducting the analysis in the cases involving patient or family requests to terminate life-sustaining treatment, various courts have asked if allowing treatment to be discontinued would violate any important state interests, including the state interest in preventing suicide. The courts consistently held that suicide was not implicated in these cases and that this presented no obstacle to acknowledging the right to refuse treatment. If such refusal was not tantamount to suicide in the eyes of the law and ethics, then what was it?

This is a familiar pattern in bioethics: medical technologies create new possibilities for human choice and action, new kinds of decisions have to be made, and a new vocabulary must be devised. Ordinary dictionary definitions are not helpful, and loose-limbed, casual talk about "wanting to die," the "right to die," and "passive and active euthanasia" has to give way to more precise, if sometimes stilted and pedantic, formulations.

Over time, those who were being careful in talking about forgoing treatment abandoned all language of suicide. They began to talk instead about the patient's right to be free of burdensome and invasive medical interventions, or the right not to have one's life prolonged by unwanted medical treatment. The proper focus is not on death but on how one lives during the course of dying. It is not death that is being chosen, but a certain form of living. Therefore, the term "right to die" is a grave misnomer. The PAS and active euthanasia arguments, on the other hand, are indeed about the right to die.

These distinctions mark something real in the experience of dying patients and their families. Thus it seems both cavalier and uncharacteristically unsophisticated for Dworkin, in his introduction to the "Philosophers' Brief," to assert that the relevant question is to distinguish "acts and omissions that are designed to cause death and those that are not," and then to combine forgoing life-sustaining treatment and PAS under the heading of acts clearly designed to cause death.[15] Dworkin continues: "In a similar vein the 'Philosophers' Brief' avers that if and when it is permissible for [a doctor] to act with death in view, it does not matter which of . . . two means he and his patient choose. If it is permissible for a doctor deliberately to withdraw medical treatment in order to allow death to result from a natural process, then it is equally permissible for him to help his patient hasten his own death more actively, if that is the patient's express wish."[16]

We should be wary of assimilating the moral significance of forgoing treatment and PAS under headings like "designed to cause death," or "with death in view," and then using that vocabulary to conclude that they are morally equivalent.

The search for an appropriate ethical and legal idiom to use in talking about medical decisionmaking near the end of life was not completed overnight, and it has had its share of missteps. Indeed, it is not yet complete. The campaign to legalize PAS continues at the level of state politics with the encouragement of the Supreme Court, which found no constitutional basis for a right to it, but also found no constitutional bar for creating a statutory right via the legislative process.

Among the dead ends that have emerged while searching for the right vocabulary have been such distinctions as "killing" versus "letting die," "acts" versus "omissions," "active euthanasia" versus "passive euthanasia," and "intending the patient's death" versus merely "foreseeing" it.

Most of these discussions boil down to questions of causation. The act versus omission distinction, preposterous on its face when applied to something like terminal and intensive medical care, has seemed promising because common sense suggests that one cannot really cause something to happen by omitting to act. Doctors do not "kill" when they only stand aside and watch. Similarly, the killing versus letting die distinction has seemed attractive because the underlying disease process, not the act of forgoing life-sustaining treatment per se, is what would really cause the patient's death.

The trouble with much of this is that there are no such things as "omissions" in the care of the dying, except if they fall under the heading of abuse and neglect, not forgoing treatment. Whether aggressive or palliative care, something is always being done with a dying patient. So there are only actions here: actions of disease modifying and life-sustaining intervention, or actions of palliative intervention, but actions nonetheless. Any of these actions can potentially bear moral (and legal) responsibility. So the connection between causation and responsibility is not nearly as straightforward as many arguments using this type of terminology—"I am not killing the patient, I am merely allowing the patient to die"—have tried to make it. Under the spell of thinking that the important difference here is in action versus nonaction, many physicians still cling to the belief that it is easier to justify morally withholding a life-sustaining treatment (e.g., a ventilator) than it is to justify withdrawing it once it has begun.

In sum, there are only actions, actions by doing and actions by forbearing to do, in the clinical care of the dying. And no one human action is *the* cause of death. Human actions and biological processes are both involved in a person's death, and rather than discovering a single cause we find multiple causal chains.

Some still cling to the hope that these causes can be fit into a rational pattern. We suggest, on the contrary, that these multiple causal chains fit together in a pattern that has the properties of a narrative rather than a scientific explanation. We cannot logically infer moral responsibility from causal explanations; instead we construct causal accounts, at least partly, on the basis of pre-established moral sensibilities and interpretations. Moral interpretation and assignment of responsibility precedes causal knowledge, not the other way around.

THE INTEGRITY OF THE PERSON AND MORAL TRESPASS

Liberal neutrality offers one way to transform medical responses to dying from a personal trouble into a civic problem. Thus far we have attempted to take stock of the paradigm shift in ethics and the law that liberal neutrality offers, particularly when it is applied to the legalization of PAS and/or active euthanasia. This shift is alluring in many ways. Perhaps, as Dworkin hopes, it offers a viable peace treaty to quell the interminable culture wars that have beset the abortion question and end-of-life issues for many years. Nonetheless, we do not believe that liberal neutrality offers the best way to frame end-of-life decisions as a civic problem. The blind spots in its perspective are too large, and its articulation of the world of the dying is inadequate.

Like all work in ethics and the law, the frame of liberal neutrality is an abstraction, a figurative construction of moral reality. It is not for this that we fault liberal neutrality, because all theoretical frameworks are figurative constructions of reality. The problem with this theory lies with what it leaves out.

What liberal neutrality obscures is the surrounding interpersonal context of the dying process. It flattens an otherwise multidimensional reality, substituting abstractions, such as "power," "control," and "interests," for entangled relationships, feelings, memories, fears, hopes, regrets, and reconciliations that admit of no such tidy characterizations.

These experiences are neither incorrigibly idiosyncratic nor wholly subjective. We feel, as we think, through publicly available concepts, categories, images, symbols, and paradigms. Without a shared culture and sustaining relationships we could not feel at all. The liberal account internalizes everything that is most social and treats it all as cognitive "beliefs" inside the head. This type of psychology is particularly debilitating when we are talking about experience at the end of life. One wonders whether it will really sustain the notion of what it is to have a belief at all, or how a dying person could tell the difference between a momentous decision and a trivial one. Respecting autonomy gives private choice value only because beyond autonomy there is a public realm of shared meaning and activity that gives each of us things of value to choose.

In short, liberal neutrality obscures crucial aspects of the human experience of dying and care giving that other conceptual frameworks can better articulate. We propose now to introduce and to emphasize two concepts that illustrate how we can go beyond the language of liberal neutrality. We refer to them as the "relational integrity of the person" and the need to protect dying persons from "moral trespass."[17]

Return for a moment to the line of cases concerning the right to forgo life-sustaining treatment. Over time two basic grounds for this right emerged. One was said to be a fundamental constitutional right of the individual to control the most important aspects of her life. In the aftermath of landmark Supreme Court rulings on reproductive rights and abortion (*Griswold*[18] and *Roe*), this right was initially associated with the concept of privacy, which the justices were then prepared to find in the Constitution. Later, especially in *Cruzan*, this was referred to as a "liberty interest" and located in the Fourteenth Amendment. In bioethics this same notion has been called individual autonomy or the right to self-determination.

The second ground for the right to refuse treatment resides in the common law as the right to be protected from nonconsensual touching (battery) or unwanted bodily invasion. The development of the law of informed consent extends that common law protection to physicians and medical care settings.

Throughout the period culminating in the *Cruzan* ruling, these two grounds were connected together in arguments in favor of such policies as advance directives, to facilitate the patient's right to refuse treatment. The movement and arguments to legalize PAS, however, drove a wedge between the autonomy and the bodily integrity notions, because the autonomy notion seems to support the contention that there is no distinction to be drawn between forgoing treatment and PAS. The bodily integrity notion, however, clearly applies to forgoing treatment but not to PAS, because in the latter it is not medical treatment or technology that is violating bodily integrity but the disease process itself. In the many amicus briefs that were filed in support of the defendants in the PAS cases, groups that formerly defended autonomy were suddenly backpedaling with vigor. Supporters of the plaintiffs, of course, stressed the continuity with earlier right-to-die rulings.

Why not simply ground the right to refuse treatment on the right to bodily integrity, and leave it at that? This is not sufficient because where autonomy tends to justify too much, bodily integrity justifies too little. For one thing, common law traditions can be superseded by statutes and do not have the same significance as constitutional rights. In an aging society it will probably be necessary to come to closure at the constitutional level. We say this with some reservation, for it is a mistake to try to turn all important questions of morality into constitutional ones. That gives undue power to the courts and suggests a lack of faith in democracy. Moreover, the concept of bodily integrity is too narrow to capture all that we want to preserve for the dying person.

What we need is a metaphorical extension of the notion of bodily integrity, one that is more focused on the surrounding relationships, the ecology of dying, and not just with the boundary of the skin. It is not simply the physical integrity of the body that we should care about but also the integrity of the person in the extended social space surrounding the physical body that makes up most of one's personhood and moral identity. This is always important, but never more so than near the end of life, when the concentric circles of one's social identity have contracted and the scope of one's active relationships have focused down to family, intimate friends, and professional caregivers.

A dying person has a right to a certain quality of living while dying, a right to a decent and nurturing social ecology. Among those things that undermine a good social ecology near the end of life, we would include uncontrolled pain, incompetent caregivers, isolation, and unwanted and intrusive medical technology. Anything that violates and undermines the social ecology of personhood constitutes a moral trespass and is an appropriate concern of bioethics, the law, and public policy.

This ecological notion of the integrity of personhood can serve as a third alternative to autonomy or self-sovereignty and to a more narrowly defined bodily integrity. Something like this notion also can be found in an undeveloped and unexplored thread of the *Quinlan* case.

QUINLAN: THE ROAD NOT TAKEN

When one rereads the text of the New Jersey Supreme Court decision *In re Quinlan* with the familiar narrative of the right-to-die debate in mind, the text is virtually incomprehensible. Whatever it may have been, this decision is certainly not simply the launch point for a journey that leads straight to the Oregon Death with Dignity Act. From the perspective of liberal neutrality, it does not talk at all about the things it should be talking about. It spends an inordinate amount of time on clearly irrelevant issues, such as the position of the Roman Catholic Church or the tradition of professional medical ethics.[19] When it mentions an "ethics committee" it seems to mean a medical prognosis committee as if some chance of recovery would override the patient's autonomous choice to forgo life-sustaining treatment.[20] It is hopelessly inconsistent as it moves back and forth between what we would now call the principle of respect for persons and the principle of beneficence or best interests.[21] It does not have a notion of substituted judgment such that it is really Karen who will make the decision through Mr. Quinlan; it seems to think that the family must be trusted and it really is Mr. Quinlan who is going to make the ultimate decision.[22] Is liberal neutrality and autonomy bioethics really already there, in embryo, preparing to gestate over the next decade into the next major cases?

We think the answer is yes and no. The seed of autonomy bioethics is there, but so is the seed of something else, something like relational integrity of the person and moral trespass. Also implicit in *Quinlan* is a different way of looking at the moral reality of the dying process.

The lessons of *In re Quinlan* remain evolving and unsettled in law and bioethics. It contains a line of reasoning about decisions near the end of life that died aborning. Both respect for autonomy and respect for relational integrity were conceptually present in the actual terminology the New Jersey Supreme Count used, namely the notion of "privacy." However, only the autonomy side of privacy has been elaborated in any systematic way by bioethics subsequent to *Quinlan*. The other idea of privacy in *Quinlan* is the idea that the rights and fundamental interests of the dying are compromised when the moral space of the person and the physical space of the body is trespassed upon not simply against one's will, but also in an inherently degrading, disruptive, and disrespectful way. This idea is the road not (yet) taken.

The idea of privacy as personal integrity involves the notion that the human good requires a defense against moral trespass of the integrity of one's person. Privacy as moral security is an ecological or relational notion not conveyed by the notions of privacy in other contexts, which involve cutting the self off from others behind protective fences.

One of the leitmotifs of *Quinlan* is the intrusive presence of machines (in particular the constantly noisy ventilator) at the bedside of the patient. Not only were these machines prolonging her dying process, they were also interfering with the kind of presence—a caring, vigilant relationship— that the family wished to have with her. The medical routines were in service to the machine, not in service to Karen, and they took precedence over the needs of the family.[23] There was no ill will or malice here. It was an ecological reality, a fact of the caregiving and grieving experience. The court had no real way to express this technological and institutional presence, this *intrusion*, but it had a recognition of it and a desire to acknowledge and ameliorate it.

The decision is also interesting for the absence of questions of conflict of interest. The court quickly dispatched such notions by establishing the guardian's and the family's character. That seems odd in light of the main issues in later cases but is perfectly understandable as a part of grounding the decision in the quality of the relationships that might surround the patient if the medical interventions did not prevent them. This made the central question not "Do I (Karen) want to die?"; nor even, "Do I want these machines?"; but rather, "How do I want to be cared for?"

Another odd aspect of the *Quinlan* decision is the serious attention the court pays to the teachings of the Quinlan family's religion, Roman Catholicism.[24] It relied heavily on an amicus brief submitted by the New Jersey Catholic Conference. The court is at pains to establish that allowing the ventilator to be removed would not violate those religious teachings.

A later attitude, and certainly the one offered by liberal neutrality, would be that this entire subject is irrelevant to the court's business. But the *Quinlan* court did not interpret this as a violation of the separation of church and state, and they were not focused on the danger of imposing some orthodox beliefs on Karen. In an uncanny prefiguring of liberal neutrality, Mr. Quinlan had asserted his right to decide his daughter's medical treatment based on his right to exercise his religion, among other grounds. The court rejected that argument, but channeled the religious question into his fitness as the guardian and how his faith would affect his relation to his daughter. Hence, the court took this question to be a vital factor in understanding the social and moral ecology of Karen's personhood, both before her brain injury and during her period of persistent vegetative state. The question of a good quality of care may include the dimension of religious and spiritual faith and practice that informs the care giving community and the care giving process, especially that of the family. An integral component of hospice services, for example, is the provision of spiritual counseling and support for both patient and family.

To be sure, the *Quinlan* court did not have the language, the metaphors, and the background in social science to formulate the question in terms like "integrity of the person," or "moral trespass." Indeed, there is no reason to think they would have embraced such language if it had been suggested to them at the time. However, our contention is that the concepts that make for the most plausible and coherent reading of their decision require something like the language of personhood and an ecology of relationships to express their meaning. Near the legal heart of the text the court makes the following statement: "We think that the State's interest [in preserving life] weakens and the individual's right to privacy grows as the degree of bodily invasion increases and the prognosis dims. Ultimately there comes a point at which the individual's right overcome the State interest. It is for that reason that we believe Karen's choice [to turn off the respirator], if she were competent to make it, would be vindicated."[25]

The first thing to notice about this formulation is that privacy is distinct from autonomy. Karen's wishes don't drive the decision, the right to privacy does. It is because Karen's wishes happen to coincide with what the right to privacy requires that the law vindicates her wishes.

The second thing to notice is that the constitutional evaluation of this situation is two-pronged: it involves medical prognosis and the "degree of bodily invasion." However, if we interpret the notion of bodily invasion narrowly (physically), then the position taken by the court is morally untenable. Assume two patients, each of whom is imminently dying. Holding that variable constant the court is saying that patient A has a greater privacy right in refusing major surgery (which is very invasive) than patient B has in refusing IV-fluids (which are minimally invasive). Surely this cannot be correct. If there is no reasonable medical purpose served by an intervention, both patients have an equally strong right to refuse it regardless of how invasive it may be. And surely the state has no greater interest in protecting the rights of one of these patients than it has in the rights of the other.

This objection is avoided if we employ the principle of interpretive charity and read the concept of "bodily integrity" in a broader and more social way. Then we can say that patients with equally grim prognoses may have different rights to the extent that their surrounding relationships and their quality of life are substantially affected by a proposed intervention. The patient does have a right to refuse entry to whatever would trespass on that care giving space, and the state does have an interest in sustaining that right (and no interest in interfering with it).

However, if a medical service arrives on the scene that does not disrupt the relational integrity surrounding the person, that has a low degree invasion of (social) bodily integrity, then it may be that the patient has a weaker right (or no right at all) to resist the intrusion of that procedure. For that entity is not an invader or a trespasser, it is just passing through. Examples of such entities might be some administrative or organizational rules of the facility that are designed for safety, efficiency, or the interests of other residents, or periodic visits by supervisors or state inspectors in home-care settings. In particular cases it may be hard to draw the line between a trespasser and a benign visitor, but that is the relevant question to ask. Things that break the patient's moral community of caring, witness, and vigil can be much worse than things that break the patient's skin.

Another peculiar thing about *Quinlan* is the way it moves back and forth between considerations that have to do with Karen's autonomy— questions of what she would want and whether this accords with what her father was proposing to do—and considerations of a seemingly more objective nature.

In the moral universe constructed by that text, respecting an individual's rights are not set in opposition to promoting the individual's good, and honoring human dignity are not simply a matter of doing whatever the patient wanted. Honoring the integrity of the person means that certain things ought not be thrust or forced upon them. In this case it means that medical technology, such as a ventilator, should not be used on a person for whom it provides no substantive benefit—someone, for example, in a permanent unconscious state such as Karen Ann Quinlan. To impose a treatment that promotes no flourishing is a wrongful imposition that breaks the "moral skin." It compromises something that should remain intact, that ought to have its integrity preserved. To initiate or continue life-sustaining medical treatment that compromises integrity in this way is to violate privacy; and the reason this is wrong is not because there is an autonomous right to die but because it is a good thing to keep one's moral skin intact until the very end.

Privacy's prohibition of moral trespass is neither subjective nor procedural; it isn't about patient preferences or desires, and it is not about who has the power and authority to make the decision. It is about what is right and what is wrong in terms of the patient's human flourishing and human good. For Karen Quinlan the time when the ventilator could promote her human flourishing had passed. Of course, that had to be confirmed, and thus the topic of medical prognosis loomed large in the case. Once it was confirmed, however, continued medical life-support became a trespass, a violation. The wrongness of this trespass has nothing to do with what Karen thought or said before her accident. (The *Quinlan* court declined to rule on whether Karen's prior statements were admissible because it considered them legally irrelevant to the decision.) The moral goal here is not primarily to act in accordance with the patient's wishes or values, although that is always important. The moral goal is to protect the person of the patient who exists—even if unconscious—as an embodied self still joined in a web of relationships of care and memory.

Privacy understood as personal autonomy stands in sharp contrast to the notion of privacy as protecting moral boundaries against trespass. For autonomy, the questions are all about the patient's prior beliefs and values, and whether those wishes have been recorded in advance directives, not about what medicine can really do and what furthers the human good. For privacy as protection against moral trespass, certain kinds of caregiving relationships are right and certain kinds are wrong, some are respectful and sustain integrity and some do not. It matters less who decides than that the decision be the morally proper one. For autonomy, it always must be the patient's own voice, either directly or indirectly heard, that matters. What that voice says doesn't matter—it may be Mrs. Helga Wanglie's voice saying, "Keep me alive," or that of Paul Brophy, Nancy Jobes, or Nancy Beth Cruzan saying, "Remove me from these unwanted treatments,"—just so long as it is the voice of the patient and no other. (The persons mentioned in this sentence were all patients in important right-to-die cases.)

Autonomy has no body, only mind; and it is mind with no surrounding moral and social space, no relationships that can be either distorted or undermined by medical technology or reinforced by the proper kind of care giving. It was that filled space—their ongoing relationship with their daughter—on which the Quinlan family focused, not on the isolated, hypothetically reconstructed will of their daughter. It would be mistaken to say that the court only focused on that dimension of the case, but it would be equally wrong to say that it focused, like later courts, solely on the patient's autonomy. It focused on both, but did not have an available language to express the difference.

In any case, one has the feeling that the *Quinlan* court sensed (and some later courts as well as many ethicists have seen) that it was in that relational space where the true Karen, severely diminished though she was, still resided as a moral entity. That relational space was worthy of protection, even at the price of foreshortening Karen's life, because it was constitutive of Karen's human good.

STAYING THE COURSE

Americans today are divided by two competing images of the moral predicament of the dying. One image is drawn from our great tradition of liberalism and civil rights. It is the image of the autonomous individual (or her surrogate) wielding fundamental moral and legal rights against the coercive, paternalistic, and restrictive power of the state. The other image is drawn from more domestic sources in our moral imaginations, what we might call, paraphrasing Michael Oakeshott, the voice of caring in the conversation of mankind.[26] This is the image of protecting the integrity of the dying person and the surrounding care-givers against moral trespass and disruption.

Medical technology has immense power to invade and distort the world of a caring community, as do government policies motivated by ideology or by market goals. Is medical care at the end of life fundamentally—and morally—about power and the struggle for control between the dying person and the state? Or is it fundamentally about organizing our support systems in such a way that our mortality will be accepted, and that the quality of the last chapter of our lives will be humane, respectful, and dignified? It is not yet clear which of these images will ultimately prevail.

To die well is to be loved, comforted, mourned, missed, and remembered. Living well in dying is a part of living well and should not be foreshortened by an act of direct euthanasia or assisted suicide. These propositions should not be seen as threats to individual liberty at the end of life. They ought be regarded rather as affirmations of the communal human condition and as tenets of moral common sense.

13

Beyond Autonomy:
Toward an Ethic of Interdependence

> For the real question is whether the brighter future is
> really always so distant. What if, on the contrary, it has
> been here for a long time already, and only our own
> blindness and weakness has prevented us from seeing it
> around us and within us, and kept us from developing it?
> —VÁCLAV HAVEL, *Open Letters*

ARGUMENTS FOR AND against placing coercive limits on individual autonomy can cite an endless series of cases and examples. The preceding chapters have offered a conceptual framework, not to put an end to such arguments or to provide a blueprint for social control, but to inform what is too often a simplistic debate with more depth and nuance.

But to what end do we use such a framework, and in the service of what moral values do we justify placing social limits on individual freedom?

This chapter explores a moral horizon beyond autonomy. In order to describe that horizon—that future that has been with us a long time already, as Havel puts it—we must turn once more to the tradition of Western liberalism, and we must consider the grounds upon which autonomy presumes to limit itself.

LOOKING BEYOND AUTONOMY
Liberalism is largely a discourse about freedom and responsibility, about individual self-determination and cultural limits, about personal autonomy and social control. In the history of the liberal tradition from the seventeenth century on, the discourse on these subjects has been reasonably balanced. It has, in the work of figures such as Locke, Montesquieu, Tocqueville, and even Mill, certainly recognized the importance of values on the

opposite side of freedom's ledger—responsibility, limits, order, and control. Indeed, as Sheldon Wolin has argued, if liberalism has emphasized the importance of freedom, it has done so not because it takes social order to be unimportant or insignificant but because it takes it to be all too prevalent, powerful, and ubiquitous.[1] In the political imagination of liberalism, order is more prone to smother than to shred, more likely to dominate than to disintegrate. (The fundamental difference between the liberal and conservative casts of mind lies precisely in this.) Thus the liberty of the individual must be shored up with legal protection, political power, and moral argument, particularly against the one locus of order that concerned the early modern liberals above all—the state.

Something began to happen to liberalism in the nineteenth century that has vastly expanded and accelerated since the early 1970s. Political liberalism has become social liberalism. The liberal idea of freedom has been given a distinctively libertarian interpretation as the concept of "autonomy." The traditional liberal suspicion about governmental control has been turned into a generalized contemporary suspicion of all forms of social or interpersonal control or restraint blocking the subjective will, the existential "projects" or the "life plans" of the self.

We have referred to this libertarian turn within liberalism as the "culture of autonomy." The culture of autonomy has emerged gradually out of the underlying forces of individualism, secularization, materialism, and rationalism that have defined modernity in the West. It has become a guiding principle and an explicit moral ideal in the ideologies of liberalism and capitalism, and it has achieved refined expression in some of the most influential works of moral philosophy, political theory, and literature since the French Revolution.

Autonomy has also penetrated deeply into our everyday lives. Too many people experience relationships as encroachments. Too many see disciplined study or activity as a straitjacket confining self-expression. Too many regard duties as millstones around their necks. In each case, the seductive voice of autonomy is whispering in their hearts. When people support public policies and social practices that maximize personal freedom of choice, no matter what the moral or financial cost to society and no matter how self-destructive the behavior, they are responding to the seduction of autonomy as well. Rejection of commitments, relationships, discipline, and duty are openly celebrated.

The culture of autonomy is prompting a cultural backlash, which began in the 1990s and is continuing today, particularly on the political right and in fundamentalist religious communities but also among liberal and progressive thinkers who often refer to themselves as "communitarians." The reaction to the terrorist attacks of September 11, 2001, temporarily cast the culture of autonomy in a dim light, but it is too early to tell how deep seated and lasting that reaction will be. Autonomy cannot simply be replaced by community or, much less, by unquestioning patriotism. The culture of autonomy calls for something much harder: a critical response that is pluralistic in outlook and pragmatic in spirit. One does not have to reject the entire liberal tradition in order to reject the culture of autonomy and the libertarian turn that liberalism has taken in America.

If the moral and social challenges America faces today (particularly in the behaviorally sensitive areas of health and medicine, social welfare, crime and drug use, education, and support for families and children) are to be met, we must recover—and articulate anew—a conception of freedom that is more civic and communal in orientation than autonomy or a libertarian conception of freedom. We must not accept the culture of autonomy on its own terms; we must confront that culture with an ethical discourse attuned to the human and moral significance of interdependence, mutuality, and reciprocity. In particular, we must explore the moral justification of state action and social coercion with a broader framework than that offered by autonomy liberalism, which is able to politically motivate and ethically justify the restriction of individual choice only in order to prevent harm to others.

In order to do this one must explore moral terrain beyond autonomy by examining other values that coexist with autonomy to make up social conditions within which human beings can flourish, realize their potential, and partake of both the individual and the common good. These other values relate to the human condition of interdependence, and they find a basis for a fabric of life together in precisely those aspects of life and experience that the culture of autonomy disdains and ignores. Foremost among those aspects are *need, vulnerability, frailty, fallibility, weakness,* and *mortality.* Autonomy forgets that the human being is incomplete without the mutuality of others.

It is from these characteristics of our selves that the social emotions first develop, and it is to them that the social emotions are primarily attuned. The vulnerability and dependence of the other call forth in us a moral response. The social emotions orient that response; they guide and sustain it. That moral response elicited by the vulnerability of others and our connectedness with them is what we have referred to as our moral common sense. It is a sense of a shared humanity and a sense of our own vulnerability and mortality; moral common sense is a sense of what we have in common with other members of the human moral community. Without these other values that pertain and respond to interdependence, autonomy alone does not provide an acceptable moral understanding of the human good, or of the fabric of our lives as moral beings. The social emotions are not symptoms of moral childishness; they are the signs of moral engagement, embeddedness, and maturity. Persons without shame, guilt, pride, and conscience are not admirable—they are morally mal-formed. That is nothing to celebrate. In a culture and social order that deliberately and systematically tries to produce such people, there is little to praise.

America today faces the paradoxical task of combining seeming oppo-sites. We must learn to use coercion for the sake of autonomy, and appeal to autonomy to reach for a form of moral life richer than the one autonomy alone can supply. Conservative critics of autonomy embrace forms of social control that penalize behavior that violates traditional moral rules. Where we differ from these critics is that we believe the power of social institutions should be used not only to deter morally wrong conduct but also to enable constructive, responsible conduct. Society not only has a right to protect the unknowing from infection, it has an obligation to do so. We have an obligation to prevent teenage pregnancies. We have an obligation to protect the mentally ill from their darker selves. And all of us as citizens have an obligation to support—and to pay for with our taxes—the institu-tions that respond to these obligations and supply the necessary services and programs.

If one is concerned about the destruction of relationships in the family, then one must also look to the corrosive, disruptive effects of the market system, as well as the perverse incentives built into the welfare state. If one is concerned about the devastating psychological effects on children of inadequate parenting and early childhood stimulation by adult caregivers, then one must promote adequate public funding and regulation for day care centers and generous corporate parental leave policies, as exist in Scandinavian countries, as well as take vigorous steps to discourage teenage pregnancy and to break the vicious cycle of multigenerational dependency on welfare support. The radical change from welfare to "workfare" long advocated by conservative policy analysts such as Charles Murray formed the basis for the 1996 Clinton welfare reforms. In eliminating the federal Aid to Families with Dependent Children (AFDC) program, the administration and Congress took the unusual step of eliminating a social right or entitlement that had been previously established, although this affected a population that is among the least well-organized, politically active, or powerful groups in our society. Whether this will be a positive step toward greater self-esteem and self-reliance for low-income women and children, or simply a harsh expression of the antigovernment and antiegalitarian ideology now dominant in national politics remains to be seen. If a coercive measure such as requiring low income beneficiaries to obtain income producing jobs within a certain period of time, on pain of loss of public benefits, is to be justified then it must demonstrably move toward the former, not the latter, goal. And it must be accompanied by the surrounding supportive measures of meaningful and effective job training, and accessible child care services that are prerequisites of any reasonable social requirement that able-bodied adults make the effort to enter the economy and become self-supporting. There is an important moral difference between asking individuals to be socially responsible and asking them to make personal tragic choices and be irresponsible parents in order to be responsible citizens.

THE HARM PRINCIPLE AND ITS LIMITS

Does autonomy provide a moral basis for its own curtailment? To some extent and in characteristically individualistic ways, it does. Autonomy does not entail the political philosophy called anarchism, although many strongly libertarian defenders of autonomy, such as Robert Paul Wolff and Robert Nozick, come close to it. Political anarchism is the doctrine that no state or government can be morally justified; social anarchism goes one step further and holds that no coercive social or cultural pressures should ever be imposed on the individual either. For anarchists, human beings are naturally free and autonomous; they have natural rights to life, liberty, and property that no social institution or majority can rightfully take away. States and governments have arisen historically to enslave people, and political power has always been imposed.

The concept of autonomy that is most influential in the United States today is an offshoot of liberalism, not anarchism. For liberals, state and social authority can be morally justified, and some means of social control can rightly override the autonomy of the individual under certain limited circumstances. Although significant in practice, the philosophical gap between liberalism and anarchism is not wide. It comes down to different empirical assumptions about what is historically likely and possible. Anarchists are optimists about human nature. They believe that people can in fact achieve voluntary and spontaneous harmony and cooperation. Crime, poverty, and other sources of conflict arise because of the unnatural and corrupting conditions created by political authority itself and its corresponding social inequality. Hence the conflict that most people think makes the state necessary is actually caused by that very remedy; abolish the state, and the need for it will wither away.

Liberals are pessimists on this score. "The latent causes of faction [conflict] are . . . sown in the nature of man," writes James Madison in *The Federalist*.[2] Liberals are prepared to accept the fact that left to their own devices, individuals will violate one another's rights. Social controls are necessary to keep interactions within the bounds of justice. The problem for liberalism, then, has been to find a moral justification for social control that adequately sustains social order, while at the same time giving individual freedom of choice, self-determination, and self-sovereignty—in a word, autonomy—as much free rein as possible.

The definitive answer to this question, for traditional liberalism and for the later culture of autonomy, was supplied by John Stuart Mill in *On Liberty*:

> One very simple principle [is] entitled to govern absolutely the dealings of society with the individual in the way of compulsion and control, whether the means used be physical force in the form of legal penalties or the moral coercion of public opinion. That principle is that the sole end for which mankind are warranted, individually or collectively, in interfering with the liberty of action

of any of their number is self-protection. That the only purpose for which power can be rightfully exercised over any member of a civilized community, against his will, is to prevent harm to others. His own good, either physical or moral, is not sufficient warrant. He cannot rightfully be compelled to do or forbear because it will be better for him to do so, because it will make him happier, because, in the opinions of others, to do so would be wise or even right. These are good reasons for remonstrating with him, or reasoning with, or persuading him, or entreating him, but not for compelling him or visiting him with any evil in case he do otherwise. To justify that, the conduct from which it is desired to deter him must be calculated to produce evil to someone else. The only part of the conduct of anyone for which he is amenable to society is that which concerns others. In the part which merely concerns himself, his independence is, of right, absolute. Over himself, over his own body and mind, the individual is sovereign.[3]

When an innocent bystander's safety, health, or well-being is endangered by an individual's behavior, autonomy can be overridden on the basis that Mill described and that contemporary philosophers now commonly refer to as the "harm principle." Preventing harm to others is virtually the only thing that can be used to justify coercive interference to limit the freedom of choice of an autonomous adult.

How does the harm principle work in practice? Not all that well. It depends on how harm is defined, who defines it, and what criteria are used. The notion of harm is not only too limiting, it can be dangerously elastic. For example, several states have so-called Megan's Laws, which requires public disclosure of the address of previously convicted sex offenders when they are released from prison and move into a community in the state. Here the notion is that the privacy of these individuals should be subordinated in order to protect the community from the harm or the threat of not knowing that a convicted sex offender or child molester is living in their midst. If we define harm this broadly, however, where would disclosure of risk stop?

Another example is provided by local ordinances in Indianapolis and in the 1982 Canadian constitution, the Charter of Rights and Freedoms.

These laws ban pornography, not on the traditional grounds that it violates community morality but on the grounds that pornographic images and speech are harmful and discriminatory per se to women. Antihate speech codes and rules on many college campuses are based on analogous notions of discrimination and harm.

Other things that on the basis of common sense might seem to be harms are not so construed by defenders of autonomy. One notorious example was the affirmation by the U.S. Supreme Court in 1978 of the right of American Nazis to march in Skokie, Illinois, a community in which many Jewish survivors of the Holocaust reside. The American Civil Liberties Union (ACLU) supported the Nazis right to march (on grounds of autonomy and freedom of expression), and the controversy nearly tore the ACLU apart. How grave does offense have to be before it becomes harm? Apparently, pictures of genitals in Indianapolis are harmful, but swastikas and brown shirts in Skokie are not.

Similarly, some would argue that the harm principle should be invoked to control that behavior of pregnant women that would adversely affect the health or well-being of the unborn fetus she intends to carry to term. When the question has been raised, however, the courts have most often come down on the side of women's autonomy rather than protection of the fetus, particularly when something of significant interest to the woman, like a well-paying job, was at stake.

Still, a commonsense morality in which responsibility supersedes autonomy remains a strong undercurrent in this highly charged area. Informal pressures abound, and various attempts to influence pregnant women's behavior continue to be made, in spite of their questionable legal status. Signs in public taverns warn pregnant women not to drink, and in some instances waiters or bartenders have refused to serve them. Social pressures and adverse reactions even from strangers are beginning to mount on pregnant women who smoke. Medical coercion and even legal sanctions were used in the drug counseling program at the prenatal clinic of the Medical University of South Carolina (discussed in chapter 9). Fearing lawsuits and avowing a concern for the unborn, some corporations have tried to adopt policies that exclude women factory workers who could not prove that they were infertile from certain high-paying jobs because they could be exposed to chemicals that would harm not their own health but that of their fetus. These policies, like the one at MUSC, have been overturned by the courts.

Real irony is inherent in those examples where the harm principle has been invoked on behalf of the unborn child. For one thing, the harm principle has an impact only on those women who choose not to exercise their autonomous legal right to abortion. The abortion debate since the *Roe v. Wade* decision of 1973 has taken place within the intellectual framework of liberal autonomy. Basically the effect of *Roe* was to hold that until the point of fetal viability, the harm principle does not apply because the previable fetus is not a person whom the Constitution (or our public morality) must protect from harm.

Opponents of legal abortion who believe that the fetus is a "person"— or at any rate a human being, a member of the human moral community and deserving of protection—could use the harm principle to override the autonomy of a woman in straightforward liberal fashion. Anti-abortion advocates sometimes do use this liberal terminology; of course, other religious and moral ideas, not all of which are compatible with liberalism, undergird their arguments as well.

Still, the framework of autonomy does give both prochoice and prolife sides of the abortion debate a common reference point. They come to opposite conclusions within the same logic of ideas because they disagree on the status of the fetus on whose behalf the harm principle is to be invoked. The harm principle does not, however, encourage discussion about the crucial effects that either allowing or banning abortion would have on the character and texture of our lives together in a moral community. Both prochoice and prolife advocates are so focused on rights that they lose sight of the world in which rights are exercised and enjoyed. The quality of the world we live in, the world that shapes us, is pushed to the periphery of the debate.

The culture of autonomy forces civic discourse and ethical argument about social control into the narrow confines of two questions. First, what is harm? How narrowly or how broadly, and how objectively or subjectively, should harm be defined? Second, when is harm really harmful? That is, should the state override people's autonomy only to protect them from harm (or risk of harm) that is involuntary, or should it also protect people from harm to which they voluntarily expose themselves?

At least the harm principle ought to have provided a bright line to indicate when individual autonomy can be overridden. It has not. People do not always recognize harm when they see it, or else they see it too readily when it is not reasonably there. Mill's "simple principle" is not so simple.

The definition of harm is a crucial question and a thorny problem for public policy. Define harm too expansively, and autonomy shrinks. How serious does harm have to be? Is it only serious physical harm or injury, or do psychological damage, pain, and suffering count as well? What is the gradation between harm, offense, annoyance, and inconvenience? Where should we draw the line?

Over time the culture of autonomy has tried to resolve these quandaries by interpreting "harm" in terms of negative liberty and negative rights. Harms are those things that encroach on my private space, those things that I don't invite in. Privacy displaces commitment, connection, and relationship. We believe that this is too one-sided. Society's power may be used to tear down walls as well as to maintain them.

There are some limitations on voluntary transactions imposed on grounds of moral standards, to be sure. However, they come under relentless assault in the culture of autonomy. Worker-protection laws limiting working hours are still on the books to protect children. Narcotic use—even use of so-called "recreational drugs"—is still a crime. This argument may soon come to be used in the fight against smoking if cigarettes are defined as "drug-delivery devices."

The winds of the harm principle in legal and public policy debates blow in many directions, some of them not so attractive for autonomy. The insurance system now confounds John Stuart Mill's distinction between other-regarding and purely self-regarding behavior. Corporations will soon begin to take a greater interest in the health-related behaviors and characteristics of their employees—diet, exercise, smoking, genetic makeup—in order to hold down their insurance costs. This interest poses a substantial threat to the privacy and autonomy of large numbers of individuals in the coming years. But it will be justified, as all abridgments of freedom must be, on the basis of protecting the rights of healthy, well-behaved, and genetically well-endowed employees against the costly profligacy and self-abuse of those who get sick and drive up health care costs.

In Pursuit of the Good

In *The Children of Light and the Children of Darkness*, Reinhold Niebuhr makes an observation that helps point us beyond autonomy liberalism and the confines of the harm principle: "The community requires liberty as much as does the individual; and the individual requires community more than bourgeois thought comprehended. Democracy can therefore not be equated with freedom. An ideal democratic order seeks unity within the conditions of freedom, and maintains freedom within the framework of order."[4] As Niebuhr is using it, the term *democracy* refers not exclusively to a form of government but also to a broader social framework and moral outlook. The term *republic* is sometimes used in this sense. It is a way of life built out of equitable rules and common purposes, and out of mutual assistance and respect. It is an environment of cultural meaning and institutional structure that has been considered by a long line of political theorists, beginning with Aristotle, to be the most appropriate setting for the pursuit and the realization of the human good.

Aristotle believed that man is a social and political animal, a *zoon politikon*, and thus is destined by nature not for autonomy but for "citizenship": that is, for membership in a civic community—"ruling and being ruled in turn . . . with a view to attaining a way of life according to goodness."[5]

We believe that Aristotle was fundamentally right about this. Such a life—the communal, interdependent life—has a distinctive rhythm. It consists of harmonizing the needs of the self with the claims of others, and the claims of the self with the needs of others. The interdependent life has characteristic vital signs. It is measured by the systole of self-assertion and the diastole of self-restraint and accommodation—the heartbeat of the body politic. The human good encompasses autonomy, but it is richer, deeper, and more nuanced than the culture of autonomy understands.

The conception of the good required to moderate the excesses of the culture of autonomy and contain it within proper boundaries is close at hand. It is implicit in our moral common sense, and it is embedded in the lives that the vast majority of ordinary Americans lead. It is embodied in the community life of our churches, synagogues, and mosques; in the voluntary and charitable activities of service organizations and civic groups; it governs the mutual adjustments and accommodations to the limitations, needs, and talents of others that make up cooperative activity in the workplace; and it regulates the give-and-take of life within families.

Appreciating the role that human interdependence plays in the good life for individuals and the ethically good society provides a guiding orientation when balancing autonomy and social control. We offer the following principles to move toward such a balance. These considerations should guide us when we evaluate specific policies and practices that limit autonomy and seek to promote the common good. They provide a moral compass as we seek the proper uses of coercion in a free society:

- A society should be so arranged that it responds to the needs and vulnerability of its members.

- A society should protect each person from violence and exploitation.

- A society should actively promote mutual assistance and socially beneficial cooperation.

- A society should give its members equal protection of the laws and a hospitable culture of equal concern and respect.

- Public policy should sustain institutions that make it possible for people to make the best use of their interdependent condition, to make shared moral life self-fulfilling and beneficial for each person as an individual.

- Policies should reform institutions and counteract concentrations of power that impede this activity.

We will be reminded that America is a heterogeneous and pluralistic society, and so it is. However, we believe that liberals have been making a serious mistake in the past few years when they have concluded that this pluralism precludes any serious consideration of the individual or the common good. These liberals think that public moral discourse must be confined to talk of rights and interests, thereby producing what Daniel Callahan, casting a jaundiced eye on it, has aptly called a pervasive "moral minimalism."[6]

We submit, on the contrary, that it is even more important, and probably easier, to have an open, explicit discussion about matters of common interest and social morality in a pluralistic society than it is in a more tightly knit, homogeneous one. African pygmies, the BaMbuti, do not have to debate abortion, capital punishment, or military conscription. These are not issues in their society. But they do not even debate issues that are issues; they do not debate whom to marry, how to share, who should hunt and who should gather, or who should do the cooking. We do. They *know* where their community and their way of life stand. We don't. Or rather, we sometimes know what we stand for at any given time, but we have to keep working at it, and we have to keep arguing. That means we have to engage, and we have to come into conflict. Autonomy as negative liberty—Brandeis's right to be let alone, or Robert Frost's "good fences make good neighbors"[7]—is not enough to sustain a civic community or a way of life in which the human good can flourish. It means we have to have a moral vocabulary substantive and rich enough to make substantive and subtle arguments with.

An ethic of interdependence highlights several things that the culture of autonomy obscures. First, it calls attention to human frailty and mortality. Robust, rugged individualism has been America's collective denial of that reality. Every human being will get sick and die. On that cold piece of granite, any adequate conception of the human good must be anchored. The human good cannot subsist outside a social environment that responds to conditions of need and vulnerability. The culture of autonomy has almost succeeded in convincing Americans that to rely on other people is a bad thing. This is asinine. The society that makes it difficult to rely on others is a folly. Such a society can be expected to allow people the "freedom" to die in the streets uncared for and alone. William Black, the homeless man whose death we discussed in chapter 1, was a citizen of that community. He died with his autonomy unsullied in a bureaucratic world of rules, rights, and indifference.

Second, interdependence reminds us that distinctive individuality, a self of one's own, actually makes no sense apart from, or in opposition to, one's attachments. Individualism is a prescriptive doctrine that idealizes the person as such, in isolation from others. One is free to esteem individuality without embracing individualism. Individuality is formed—from infancy onward—out of the proper human interactions. And it continues through-out adult life, for the process of identity formation is both perpetually unfinished and inextricably social.

Moreover, we now all live in a society marked by increasing, not decreasing, interconnection and mutual reliance. Each of our lives is affected by more people than ever before. We generally need the cooperation of more people than ever to accomplish even those goals we set for ourselves. This insight needs no elaborate demonstration; one is reminded of it with every smoggy breath we take, and every time we step on an airplane and ponder how our life depends on the competent, attentive behavior of dozens of strangers, from the pilot to the air traffic controller to the ground mechanic who was supposed to inspect the extent of the metal fatigue on the wings. Technology increases the links that tie people together, voluntarily or not, and the complexity of our economic system and the organizations we work for multiplies these linkages.

What can autonomy as self-mastery or self-sovereignty possibly mean under such circumstances? One thing is clear: whatever self-mastery means today, it cannot be thought of as something that a person can achieve on his or her own. That sounds paradoxical, but it really is not. To exercise control over what happens to you as an individual, you must be involved with others in a process that decides what happens to you and your fellow citizens collectively. We can no longer separate the quality of personal life from the quality of social life. To preserve private space, we must also preserve the commons.

That is one reason why even in a society so seduced by and attached to autonomy, many people are now getting fed up with what can only be called acts of vandalism against the public space. Threatening, disrespectful, wanton, and manifestly selfish acts—from the warfare of crack dealers and gangs to the shameless greed of corporate, white-collar criminals who rob people of their savings and their pensions to the destruction of our very environment by industrial polluters—are poisonous to everyone, not just those directly harmed. Of course, we pay for such things as taxpayers and as consumers, but that is not the most important cost. All of us are *morally* impoverished by these assaults on the quality and integrity of our common life.

Individual self-mastery is meaningless unless we also have (or can regain, for to a great extent it has been lost) collective or civic self-mastery. Private autonomy and active democratic citizenship have been put at odds by a way of thinking that understands citizenship mainly in terms of personal rights, protections, and guarantees. The culture of autonomy has forgotten that citizenship also imposes civic obligations and requires civic virtues. Civic virtues are in fact the traits of character that make one effective in cooperative and collaborative activity and that make one at once self-respecting and respectful of others.

Consider what can happen when a climate of civic concern breaks down and gives way to a situation radically polarized by self-interest, suspicion, and hostile defensiveness. The AIDS epidemic, of course, is one of the major tragedies of our time, but it is also unfortunately a mirror of our civic condition. Earlier and more coercive public health measures in the mid-1980s could have limited the spread of AIDS. We knew how the virus was transmitted biologically and ways to control it; in the culture of autonomy we could not find a satisfactory way of controlling it politically. The debate focused almost exclusively on the evils of discrimination, and in this instance public fear of disease was not able to unleash the harm principle in the service of coercive measures such as closing of bathhouses or mandatory testing and contact tracing. Nondiscrimination and privacy are important values, but they were not the only things that needed to be discussed. There was insufficient debate on the nature of the *society* that would follow each of the two alternative approaches—libertarian or communitarian. In the end, the libertarian position might well have still carried the day over a more communitarian public health position, but the debate was not even joined clearly in those terms at the time. Only in hindsight has it been possible to articulate what was at stake beyond the immediate interest group positions, and even now that articulation remains controversial.

A society informed by an ethic of interdependence must ensure for its individual members equal protection under law in a hospitable culture. Public policy should, in addition, sustain institutions that make it possible for people to make positive use of their interdependent lives and condition, both by providing care for one another and by taking responsibility to protect others when one is in a position, due to power or contagious infection, to harm them. Policies should reform institutions and counteract concentrations of power that impede the provision of this care or the exercise of this responsibility.

Turning to a final example, we must be particularly vigilant in sustaining and protecting the institutions of socialization and character formation—both formal and informal. These institutions create what the ancient Greeks called *paideia*. By this word they meant the moral climate or temperament of the entire society, the well from which each individual drinks to sustain his principled moral commitments, and the underground spring from which each person draws, as by osmosis, his moral behavior and conscience. Without healthy institutions of socialization—families, extended kinship networks, settings of adult support and role modeling—no civilization can reproduce itself; no moral order can be passed on. We must rear children with the capacities and motivation to carry on this vocation. However crucial autonomy may be in the relationship between the individual and the state, it cannot be allowed to contribute to the unraveling of these institutions.

Here is where we must devote our energies and resources: to the breakdown of the family; to the separation of paternity from fatherhood; to children increasingly being born to children; and to those parental children increasingly becoming drug addicts. Given such perverse conditions, human nature will not produce a truly human culture, our innate potential for nobility will remain unrealized, our energies will be channeled into destructive directions, and we cannot expect the emergence of a generation of responsible adults—unless we are prepared to intervene.

How and when should society exert its efforts to contain this cycle of self-destruction? By the time the damage is evident, it is usually too late to make amends. The adolescent psychopath is the hard case that will almost always resist any treatment. That being so, then it would seem prudent, if depressing, to acknowledge our limitations and save the money for better purposes. Contain and control the psychopaths as compassionately as one can; psychiatric intervention has rarely proved of any benefit here. But attend to the very young; here we have real leverage, and their neglect will cost them and us dearly. By caring for the very young, we will diminish the future generations of antisocial misfits. We will establish the conditions that alone encourage the development of hope, identification, and the conscience necessary to enter the mainstream of society.

Children who are left untended and unloved will become the next generation of disaffected and antisocial teenagers. We would be wise to devote our primary energies and the bulk of our funds to preventing that from happening. The interventions need not be draconian—most impoverished parents would welcome such programs with open arms.

The model of available free public education ought to be extended into infancy. Here we need no highly expensive trained professionals like psychologists or psychiatrists. Communities have untapped human resources, where the time and experience of an older generation could supply true caring and nurture for the neglected preschool child. They could supply the models. They could form a bridge from one generation to another. They could repair the social fabric.

Low-cost day care centers could function with caring older women in the community, who could use the employment opportunities. They need have no special skills beyond a caring nature. We must resist the tendency to "civilize" children or even "educate" them. All that infants require to mature into humane adults is the simplest administration of touching, feeling, caring, and loving. Nature will do the rest for us, gratis. If these programs are important enough to create, and they are, they are important enough to make mandatory for infants who would otherwise be denied the crucial early nurturing so vital for later social development. This area is sufficiently crucial to *coerce* compliance. Mandatory neonatal and infant care is as important for the moral community as mandatory education is for the social community.

Of course, some will see this as an infringement of the autonomous rights of the teenage parent. The concept of mandatory education was also once perceived as an infringement on parental rights. We will have to weigh the autonomous rights of the mother against the anticipated benefits to the child and the society at large. The sociopathic behavior that results when a child is deprived of the care and attention, the love and concern, that are his due during his years of dependence is the punishment we will continue to suffer for our selfish neglect of these children. In contrast, by mandating caring we will offer the now-deprived child a precious gift: the gift of pride and belonging. Pride and belonging give freedom of choice value because they give a person something of value to choose.

REIMAGINING FREEDOM, REMEMBERING SOCIETY

In Gordon Wood's magnificent interpretation of the American Revolution he, like Tocqueville before him, sees the problems of individualism as endemic to the logic of modern democracy, of which America has been, thus far, the purest example. He views democratic individualism and equality as the primary and most radical achievement of the revolution, but he also argues that this equality brought with it a deep suspicion of all authority. And it laid the groundwork for a conflict among different essential principles of democracy, none of which ought be sacrificed for any other. Wood closes his book with an affirmation of American democracy to which we heartily subscribe: "No doubt the cost that America paid for this democracy was high—with its vulgarity, its materialism, it rootlessness, its anti-intellectualism. But there is no denying the wonder of it and the real earthly benefits it brought to the hitherto neglected and despised masses of common laboring people. The American Revolution created this democracy, and we are living with its consequences still."[8]

Dostoyevsky's Grand Inquisitor was convinced that the burden of freedom and moral responsibility was too heavy for human beings to bear, and that it was necessary to choose between order and happiness on the one side, and freedom on the other. For the Inquisitor, the problems we have wrestled with in this book would be easy to solve. Fortunately our predicament is richer, but also more inescapable, than his.

Our society stands poised between two compelling moral visions. One is the deeply moving transformation that Baby Suggs and Sethe experienced when they finally felt the gravity of freedom and the meaning of being a person in oneself and for oneself. The other is the promise of civic community and mutuality that courses through the Western political tradition.

America stands poised there, and perhaps that is not such a bad place to be. It is time for all of us to respond to Václav Havel's challenge to "reflect concretely on our own experience and to give some thought to whether certain elements of that experience do not—without our really being aware of it—point somewhere further, beyond their apparent limits."[9] We are firm in our belief that these two visions of freedom and community can hold together. The social and moral imagination necessary to sustain the proper balance and creative tension between them is available in contemporary America. We must join together in using that imagination.

Notes

Chapter 1. Freedom, Coercion, and Commonsense Morality

1. N. K. Kleinfield, "Everyone Followed the Rules, but a Man Died," *New York Times*, 23 October 1994, 37–38.

2. J. B. Schneewind, *The Invention of Autonomy: A History of Modern Moral Philosophy* (Cambridge: Cambridge University Press, 1998).

3. Christopher Lasch, *The Culture of Narcissism* (New York: Norton, 1975); Charles Taylor, *The Ethics of Authenticity* (Cambridge, Mass.: Harvard University Press, 1991); Robert N. Bellah, Richard Madsen, William M. Sullivan, Ann Swidler, and Steven M. Tipton, *Habits of the Heart: Individualism and Commitment in American Life* (Berkeley: University of California Press, 1985); and Alan Wolfe, *Moral Freedom: The Search for Virtue in a World of Choice* (New York: Norton, 2001).

4. *Moral Freedom*, 195.

5. Ibid., 198.

6. David Riesman, Nathan Glazer, and Reuel Denney, *The Lonely Crowd: A Study of the Changing Amnerican Character* (New Haven, Conn.: Yale University Press, 1950); Robert N. Bellah, Richard Madsen, William M. Sullivan, Ann Swidler, and Steven M. Tipton, *Habits of the Heart: Individualism and Commitment in American Life* (Berkeley: University of California Press, 1985); E. J. Dionne, Jr., *Why Americans Hate Politics* (New York: Simon and Schuster, 1991).

7. Claudia Dreifus, "Joycelyn Elders," *Sunday New York Times Magazine*, 30 January 1994, 18.

8. Jose Delgado, *The Physical Control of the Mind* (New York: Harper and Row, 1969).

9. Vernon Mark and Frank Ervin, *Violence and the Brain* (New York: Harper and Row, 1970).

10. Willard Gaylin, "The Frankenstein Factor," *New England Journal of Medicine* 297 (September 22, 1977): 665.

11. Robert Pear, "Serious Troubles are Found in Federal Vaccine Program," *New York Times*, 17 July 1994, 16.

12. Ibid.

Chapter 2. A Self of One's Own

1. Tom Beauchamp and James Childress, *Principles of Biomedical Ethics*, 4th ed. (New York: Oxford University Press, 1994), 121.

2. Thomas Scanlon, "A Theory of Freedom of Expression," *Philosophy and Public Affairs* 1 (1972): 215.

3. Robert Paul Wolff, *In Defense of Anarchism* (New York: Harper and Row, 1970), 14.

4. R. S. Peters, "Freedom and the Development of the Free Man," in *Education and the Development of Reason*, ed. R. F. Dearden (London: Routledge and Kegan Paul, 1972), 130.

5. See Lawrence Kohlberg, *Essays on Moral Development*, vol. 1: *The Philosophy of Moral Development* (New York: Harper and Row, 1981).

6. Lawrence Haworth, *Autonomy* (New Haven, Conn.: Yale University Press, 1986), 46.

7. Joel Feinberg, "The Idea of a Free Man," in *Education and the Development of Reason*, ed. R. F. Dearden (London: Routledge and Kegan Paul), 161.

8. In describing the historical and ideological background to modern liberalism, we have found the following works particularly instructive: Quentin Skinner, *The Foundations of Modern Political Thought*, 2 volumes (Cambridge: Cambridge University Press, 1978); J. G. A. Pocock, *The Machiavellian Moment: Florentine Political Thought and the Atlantic Republican Tradition* (Princeton, N.J.: Princeton University Press, 1975); Nannerl O. Keohane, *Philosophy and the State in France: The Renaissance to the Enlightenment* (Princeton, N.J.: Princeton University Press, 1980); Charles Taylor, *Sources of the Self: The Making of the Modern Identity* (Cambridge, Mass.: Harvard University Press, 1989).

9. Giovanni Pico della Mirandola, "Oration on the Dignity of Man," in *Classics of Western Thought*, vol. 2, ed. Karl F. Thompson (New York: Harcourt Brace Jovanovich, 1973), 204.

10. Donald J. Wilcox, *In Search of God and Self: Renaissance and Reformation Thought* (Boston: Houghton Mifflin, 1975).

11. Galatians 3:23–25.

12. Galatians 5:13–15.

13. Max Weber, *The Protestant Ethic and the Spirit of Capitalism*, trans. Talcott Parsons (New York: Charles Scribner's Sons, 1958).

14. Archibald MacLeish quoted in Alan Brinkley, "For America, It Truly Was a Great War," *Sunday New York Times Magazine*, 7 May 1995, 57.

15. Ralph Waldo Emerson, *Essays and Lectures* (New York: Library of America, 1983), 261.

16. Toni Morrison, *Beloved* (New York: Penguin, 1988), 141.

17. See John Rawls, *A Theory of Justice* (Cambridge, Mass.: Harvard University Press, 1971); and Ronald Dworkin, "Liberalism," in *Public and Private Morality*, ed. Stuart Hampshire (New York: Cambridge University Press, 1978), 113–43. For a discussion of what Rawls refers to as the "thin theory of the good," see Michael J. Sandel, *Liberalism and the Limits of Justice* (New York: Cambridge University Press, 1982).

18. William Blake, "London," from *Complete Writings*, ed. Geoffrey Keynes (New York: Oxford University Press, 1969), 216.

19. Morrison, *Beloved*, 162.

20. Molière, *The Misanthrope*, trans. Richard Wilbur, in *The Classic Theatre*, ed. Eric Bentley (New York: Anchor Books, 1961), 66–69.

21. Isaiah Berlin, *Four Essays on Liberty* (New York: Oxford University Press, 1969), 127.

22. *Olmsted v. United States*, U.S. 438, 478 (1928).

23. Berlin, *Four Essays on Liberty*, 131.

24. Joel Feinberg, "The Nature and Value of Rights," in *Rights, Justice, and the Bounds of Liberty*, ed. Joel Feinberg (Princeton, N.J.: Princeton University Press, 1980), 143–58.

Chapter 3. Land of the Free

1. Mary Ann Glendon, *Rights Talk: The Impoverishment of Political Discourse* (New York: Free Press, 1991).

2. Denis Johnson, "The Militia in Me," *Esquire* 124: 1 (July 1995), 40.

3. Gordon S. Wood, *The Radicalism of the American Revolution* (New York: Vintage Books, 1991), 308.

4. Ibid.

5. *Olmstead v. United States*, U.S. 438, 478 (1928).

6. Bruce Ackerman, *Social Justice in the Liberal State* (New Haven, Conn.: Yale University Press, 1980), 368–69.

7. Johnson, "Militia in Me," 40.

8. See Henry Kamm, "In Prosperous Singapore, Even the Elite Are Nervous about Speaking Out," *New York Times*, 13 August 1995, 10.

9. Owen Fiss, "Groups and the Equal Protection Clause," in *Equality and Preferential Treatment*, ed. Marshall Cohen, Thomas Nagel, and Thomas Scanlon (Princeton, N.J.: Princeton University Press, 1977), 84–154.

10. On this complicated issue generally, see Aaron Wildavsky, *But Is It True?: A Citizen's Guide to Environmental Health and Safety Issues* (Cambridge, Mass.: Harvard University Press, 1995), 55–80.

11. Daniel Yankelovich, *New Rules: Searching for Self-Fulfillment in a World Turned Upside Down* (New York: Random House, 1981), 9.

12. Ibid., xviii.

13. Joseph Berger, "Discrimination or Discourtesy?: A Commuter Won't Leave Her Bus Seat for Hasidic Prayer Meeting," *New York Times*, 9 September 1994, B1.

14. Joseph Berger, "Commuters Reach Settlement over Jewish Prayers on Bus," *New York Times*, 14 March 1995, B4.

15. James Q. Wilson, *The Moral Sense* (New York: Free Press, 1994), 234.

Chapter 4. Seduced by Autonomy

1. Stanley Hauerwas, *Vision and Virtue* (Notre Dame, Ind.: Fides Publishers, 1974); Daniel Bell, *The Cultural Contradictions of Capitalism* (New York: Basic Books, 1976).

2. Robert Hughes, *Culture of Complaint: The Fraying of America* (New York: Oxford University Press, 1993).

3. Jean Bethke Elshtain, *Democracy on Trial* (New York: Basic Books, 1995).

4. William A. Henry III, *In Defense of Elitism* (New York: Doubleday, 1994).

5. Philip K. Howard, *The Death of Common Sense: How Law Is Suffocating America* (New York: Random House, 1994).

6. Gertrude Himmelfarb, *The De-Moralization of Society: From Victorian Virtues to Modern Values* (New York: Alfred A. Knopf, 1995); and Arthur M. Schlesinger, Jr., *The Disuniting of America* (New York: W. W. Norton, 1992).

7. Philip P. Hallie, *Lest Innocent Blood Be Shed: The Story of the Village of Le Chambon and How Goodness Happened There* (New York: Harper and Row, 1979).

8. John Donne, "An Anatomie of the World" (lines 205, 213–18), in *The Complete Poetry and Selected Prose of John Donne*, ed. Charles M. Coffin (New York: Random House, 1952), 191.

9. William Shakespeare, *Troilus and Cressida*, Act I, Scene 3.

10. See Arthur O. Lovejoy, *The Great Chain of Being* (New York: Harper and Row, 1960 [1936]); and E. M. W. Tillyard, *The Elizabethan World Picture* (New York: Random House, n.d.).

11. Fyodor Dostoevsky, *The Brothers Karamazov*, trans. Richard Pevear and Larissa Volokhonsky (New York: Random House, 1990), 254–55.

12. Ibid., 258.

Chapter 5. It's Only Human Nature

1. Theodosius Dobzhansky, *Mankind Evolving* (New Haven, Conn.: Yale University Press, 1962), 346–47.

2. Genesis 2:16–17.

3. Immanuel Kant, *On History*, ed. L. W. Beck (New York: Bobbs-Merrill, 1963), 55.

4. Genesis 2:16–17.

5. Jean-Jacques Rousseau, *The First and Second Discourses*, ed. R. D. Masters (New York: St. Martin's Press, 1964), 113–15.

6. Ibid., 114–15.

7. Julian Huxley, *Man in the Modern World* (New York: Mentor Books, 1944), 16–17.

8. Stephen Jay Gould, *Ever Since Darwin: Reflections in Natural History* (New York: W. W. Norton, 1977), pp. 79–90.

Chapter 6. Growing Up Good

1. Sigmund Freud, *Totem and Taboo*, trans. James Strachey (New York: W. W. Norton, 1950), 126–46.

2. Adolf Portmann, *Animals as Social Beings* (New York: Harper and Row, 1964), 75–76.

3. Ambrose Bierce, *The Devil's Dictionary*, (1911; reprint, New York: Dover, 1993), 46.

4. See M. Kurlansky, *The Soul of Graffiti*. Documented by M. Kurlansky and J. Naar. Text by Norman Mailer (New York: Praeger, 1974).

Chapter 7. Irrational Man

1. William Barrett, *Irrational Man* (New York: Doubleday Anchor, 1962), 278–79.

2. Romans 7:13.

3. Gina Kolata, "Advice Unheeded on Averting Birth Defect," *New York Times*, 4 March 1995, 7.

4. B. F. Skinner, *Beyond Freedom and Dignity* (New York: Alfred A. Knopf, 1971).

5. For an expanded discussion of human dependence, see Willard Gaylin, *Caring* (New York: Alfred A. Knopf, 1976).

6. Stephen Crane, *The Red Badge of Courage* (1895; reprint, New York: Library of America, 1984).

7. See Willard Gaylin, *The Killing of Bonnie Garland* (New York: Penguin Books, 1995).

8. Paul Ricoeur, "Guilt, Ethics and Religion," in *Conscience: Theological and Psychological Perspectives*, ed. C. Nelson (New York: Newman Press, 1973), 15.

9. Aristotle, *Rhetoric* 1383b, in *Basic Works of Aristotle*, ed. R. McKeon, trans. W. Rhys Roberts (New York: Random House, 1941), 1392.

10. Aristotle, *Rhetoric* 1384a, in *Basic Works*, 1393, emphasis added.

11. Nathaniel Hawthorne, *The Scarlet Letter* (New York: Washington Square Press, 1955), 85, 86.

12. For a more detailed discussion of the shaping of male character, see Willard Gaylin, *The Male Ego* (New York: Viking Penguin, 1992).

13. Gary Alan Fine, *With the Boys: Little League Baseball and Preadolescent Culture* (Chicago: University of Chicago Press, 1987).

14. Ovid, *Metamorphoses*, trans. Frank J. Miller, Loeb Classical Library (New York: G. P. Putnam's Sons, 1916), 1: 7.

15. Sigmund Freud, *Group Psychology and the Analysis of the Ego* (New York: Boni and Liveright, 1921), 18: 111.

Chapter 8. The Multiple Meanings of Coercion

1. *Black's Law Dictionary*, 5th ed. (St. Paul, Minn.: West Publishing, 1979), 234.

2. All definitions are from *The American Heritage Dictionary of the English Language*, 3d ed. (New York: Houghton Mifflin, 1992).

3. Jason DeParle, *New York Times*, 22 June 1994, A-16.

4. William James, "The Moral Philosopher and the Moral Life." In *The Writings of William James*, ed. J. McDermott (New York: Random House, 1967), 618–19.

5. For coercion as a crime, see NewYork Penal Law Art. 13.60 (5). For coercion as a defense, see *Haynes v. Washington* 373 U.S. 503, 1963.

6. Quoted in Paul Trachman, "NIH Looks at the Implausible and the Inexplicable," *Smithsonian* 25: 6 (September 1994), 110.

7. Richard Condon, *The Manchurian Candidate* (1959; reprint, New York: Armchair Detective, 1991).

8. As quoted in Robert Lifton, "The Revolutionary College," in *Psychiatry and Public Affairs*, Group for the Advancement of Psychiatry (Hawthorne, N.Y.: Aldine, 1966), 251.

9. Joe McGinniss, *The Selling of the President* (New York: Trident Press, 1969).

Chapter 9. In Defense of Social Control

1. Kevin Phillips, *The Politics of Rich and Poor: Wealth and the American Electorate in the Reagan Aftermath* (New York: Random House, 1990); and Phillips, *Wealth and Democracy: A Political History of the American Rich* (New York: Broadway Books, 2002), 108–70.

2. W. B. Yeats, "The Second Coming," *The Collected Poems* (New York: Macmillan, 1956), 184–85.

3. A large philosophical literature exists on the topic of coercion. The monumental work of Joel Feinberg, *The Moral Limits of the Criminal Law*, 4 vols. (New York: Oxford University Press, 1984–88), is indispensable for a serious study of the topic. Other important works include Alan Wertheimer, *Coercion* (Princeton: Princeton University Press, 1987); and J. R. Pennock and John W. Chapman, eds., *Coercion*, Nomos XIV (Chicago: Aldine, Atherton, 1972). An overview of the subject that we have found helpful is Michael R. Rhodes, "Coercion: A Nonevaluative Approach" (Ph.D. diss., State University of New York at Buffalo, 1994).

4. Thomas Hobbes, *Leviathan*, chap. XIII, ed. C. B. MacPherson (1651; Reprint: Hammonsworth, UK: Penguin, 1968), 183–88.

5. Lewis Carrol, *Alice in Wonderland* (1865; reprint, New York: Signet, 2000).

6. Colin Turnbull, *The Mountain People* (New York: Simon and Schuster, 1972).

7. Elie Halévy, *The Growth of Philosophic Radicalism* (Boston: Beacon Press, 1955).

8. Stephen Crane, *The Red Badge of Courage* (1895; reprint, New York: Library of America, 1984).

9. Mark Twain, *Adventures of Huckleberry Finn* (1876; reprint, New York: Library of America, 1982).

10. Robert D. Putnam, *Bowling Alone: The Collapse and Revival of American Community* (New York: Simon and Schuster, 2000); and Stephen Baron, John Field, and Tom Schuller, eds. *Social Capital: Critical Perspectives* (New York: Oxford University Press, 2000).

11. Robert Nozick, "Coercion," in P. Laslett, W. G. Runciman, and Q. Skinner, eds., *Philosophy, Politics, and Society*, 4th series (Oxford: Basil Blackwell, 1972), 101–35; and Joseph Raz, *The Morality of Freedom* (Oxford: Oxford University Press, 1979), 148–57.

12. Stephen Jay Gould, "So Near and Yet So Far," *New York Review of Books* 41:17 (October 20, 1994), 24–28.

13. William Styron, *Sophie's Choice* (1976; reprint, New York: Modern Library, 2000).

14. John Stuart Mill, *On Liberty*, ed. C. V. Shields (1859; reprint, Indianapolis, Ind.: Bobbs-Merrill, 1956).

15. *Ferguson et al. v. City of Charleston et al.*, 532 U.S. 67, 121 S. Ct. 1281 2001.

16. Timothy Egan, "When Young Break the Law, a Town Charges the Parents," *New York Times*, 31 May 1995, A-1, B-7.

Chapter 10. Autonomy Gone Bonkers

1. E. Fuller Torrey, *Nowhere to Go: The Tragic Odyssey of the Homeless Mentally Ill* (New York: Harper and Row, 1981).

2. Christopher Jencks, *The Homeless* (Cambridge, Mass.: Harvard University Press, 1994).

3. Nancy Rhoden, "The Limits of Liberty: Deinstitutionalization, Homelessness, and Libertarian Theory," *Emory Law Journal* 31: 2 (spring 1982): 375–440.

4. A. Arce and M. J. Vergare, "Identifying and Characterizing the Mentally Ill among the Homeless," in *The Homeless Mentally Ill*, ed. H. R. Lamb (Washington, D.C.: American Psychiatric Association, 1984), 77.

5. Jencks, *Homeless*, 13.

6. As reported in R. White, *Rude Awakenings: What the Homeless Crisis Tells Us* (San Francisco: Institute for Contemporary Studies, 1992), 3.

7. Jencks, *Homeless*, 102.

8. Norman Q. Brill, "Deinstitutionalization," *American Journal of Social Psychiatry* 3 (summer 1985): 54.

9. Rhoden, "Limits," 380.

10. Thomas Szasz, *The Myth of Mental Illness: Foundations of a Theory of Personal Conduct* (New York: Hoeber-Harper, 1961).

11. Andrew Scull, *Decarceration, Community Treatment and the Deviant: A Radical View* (Englewood Cliffs, N.J.: Prentice Hall, 1977).

12. M. Plott, "Man Who Blinded Self Is Moved from Prison," *Atlanta Constitution*, 8 March 1985, as quoted in Torrey, *Nowhere to Go*, 12.

13. Rhoden, "Limits," 377.

14. Jencks, *Homeless*, 29.

15. Ibid., 32

16. P. Applebaum and T. Gutheil, "The Boston State Hospital Case," *American Journal of Psychiatry* 137 (1980): 720–23.

17. As reported in Torrey, *Nowhere to Go*, 9.

18. "For Some Mentally Ill, Road to Treatment Begins in Jail," *Erie Alliance for the Mentally Ill Newsletter* (March 1987), as quoted in Torrey, *Nowhere to Go*, 11.

19. Jencks, *Homeless*, 120.

20. Henri Bergson, *Time and Free Will* (London: George Allen and Unwin, 1910), 172. We have modified the translation somewhat.

21. Nigel Walker, *Crime and Insanity in England* (Edinburgh, Scotland: Edinburgh University Press, 1968), 63.

Chapter 11. Last Rights I: Decisions to Forgo Life-Sustaining Medical Treatment

1. Carl E. Schneider, *The Practice of Autonomy: Patients, Doctors, and Medical Decisions* (New York: Oxford University Press, 1998).

2. This tendency toward overly aggressive end-of-life care has been documented thoroughly by a massive study of the care of patients believed to have less than six months to live at several major medical centers. Cf., SUPPORT Principal Investigators, "A Controlled Trial to Improve Care for Seriously Ill Hospitalized Patients: The Study to Understand Prognoses and Preferences for Outcomes and Risks of Treatments (SUPPORT)," *Journal of the American Medical Association* 274 (1995): 1591–98.

3. *Cruzan v. Director, Missouri Department of Health*, 110 S. Ct. 2841 (1990).

4. 42 USC, §§ 1395cc, 1396a.

5. President's Commission for the Study of Ethical Problems in Medicine and Biomedical and Behavioral Research, *Deciding to Forego Life-Sustaining Treatment* (Washington, D.C.: Government Printing Office, 1983), 43–44.

6. John Donne, *Devotions upon Emergent Occasions*, "Meditation XVII," in *The Complete Poetry and Selected Prose of John Donne*, ed. Charles M. Coffin (New York: Random House, 1952), 441: "No man is an Iland, intire of it selfe; every man is a peece of the Continent, a part of the maine: . . . any mans death diminishes me, because I am involved in Mankinde; And therefore never send to know for whom the bell tolls; It tolls for thee."

7. Cf., The Hastings Center, *Guidelines on the Termination of Life Sustaining Treatment and the Care of the Dying* (Bloomington: Indiana University Press, 1987); and National Center for State Courts, *Guidelines for State Court Decision Making in Life Sustaining Medical Treatment Cases*, 2d ed. (Williamsburg, Va.: National Center for State Courts, 1992); See also, The New York State Task Force on Life and the Law, *When Others Must Choose: Deciding for Patients without Capacity* (Albany, N.Y.: Health Re-

search, 1992); and Alan Meisel, "Forgoing Life Sustaining Treatment: The Legal Consensus," *Kennedy Institute of Ethics Journal* 2:4 (December 1992).

8. Cf. Ezekiel J. Emanuel, *The Ends of Human Life: Medical Ethics in a Liberal Polity* (Cambridge, Mass.: Harvard University Press, 1991), 42–96. See also Nancy Rhoden, "Litigating Life and Death," *Harvard Law Review* 102 (1988): 375–446.

9. *In re Martin*, 450 Mich. 204; 538 N.W.2d 399 (1995).

10. *Wendland v. Wendland*, 26 Cal. 4th 519, 28 P.3d 151 (2001). For a discussion, see Bernard Lo, Laurie Dornbrand, Leslie E. Wold, and Michelle Groman, "The Wendland Case: Withdrawing Life Support from Incompetent Patients Who Are Not Terminally Ill," *New England Journal of Medicine* 346, no. 19 (May 9, 2002): 1489–93.

11. Nancy Rhoden, "Litigating Life and Death," *Harvard Law Review* 102 (1988): 437–45.

12. John Hardwig, "What about the Family?" *Hastings Center Report* 20, no. 2 (1990): 5–10.

13. James Lindemann Nelson, "Taking Families Seriously," *Hastings Center Report* 22, no. 4 (1992): 6–12.

14. Charles Taylor, *The Ethics of Authenticity* (Cambridge, Mass.: Harvard University Press, 1991).

15. A notable example is Joseph Raz, *The Morality of Freedom* (New York: Oxford University Press, 1986). For a general discussion of liberalism and the good see William Galston, *Liberal Purposes* (Cambridge: Cambridge University Press, 1991); and Rogers Smith, *Liberalism and American Constitutional Law* (Cambridge, Mass.: Harvard University Press, 1985).

Chapter 12. Last Rights II: Autonomy, Moral Trespass, and Physician-Assisted Suicide

1. The literature on liberal neutrality is quite large and growing. For a recent overview and critique see George Sher, *Beyond Neutrality* (Princeton, N.J.: Princeton University Press, 1997). Bioethics, the law, liberal neutrality, and death and dying all come together in one fascinating text: the so-called "Philosophers' Brief," an amicus brief to the U.S. Supreme Court concerning the PAS cases. Cf. Brief for Ronald Dworkin et al., as Amicus Curiae Supporting Respondent, *Vacco v. Quill*, 521 U.S. 793 (1997). Reprinted as Ronald Dworkin, Thomas Nagel, Robert Nozick, John Rawls, Thomas Scanlon, and Judith Jarvis Thomson, "Assisted Suicide: the Philosophers' Brief," *New York Review of Books*, 44 (March 27, 1997), 41–47.

2. 355 A.2d 647 (N.J. 1976).

3. SUPPORT Principal Investigators, "A Controlled Trial to Improve Care for Seriously Ill Hospitalized Patients: The Study to Understand Prognoses and Preferences for Outcomes and Risks of Treatments (SUPPORT)," *Journal of the American Medical Association* 274 (1995): 1591–98.

4. 97 F.3d 708 (2d Cir. 1996) rev'd *Vacco v. Quill*, 521 U.S. 793 (1997).

5. 79 F.3d 790 (9th Cir. 1996), rev'd *Washington v. Glucksberg et al.*, 521 U.S. 702 (1997).

6. The Oregon Death With Dignity Act, Ore. Rev. Stat. 127.800, 127.805 (1996).

7. C. Wright Mills, *The Sociological Imagination* (New York: Oxford University Press, 1959), 8–9.

8. Ronald Dworkin, *Life's Dominion* (New York: Knopf, 1993).

9. Ibid., 181–82.

10. Ibid., 157–59.

11. 410 U.S. 113 (1973).

12. "Assisted Suicide: The Philosophers' Brief," *New York Review of Books* 44 (March 27, 1997), 41.

13. Ibid., 43.

14. 505 U.S. 883 (1992): "Matters involving the most intimate and personal choices a person may make in a lifetime, choices central to a person's dignity and autonomy, are central to the liberty protected by the Fourteenth Amendment," at 851.

15. "Philosophers' Brief," 42.

16. Ibid., 45.

17. The term "trespass" and indeed much of the notion of the relational integrity of the person was suggested to us by Paul Ramsey, *The Patient as Person* (New Haven, Conn.: Yale University Press, 1970), xiii: "Just as man is a *sacredness in the social and political order*, so he is a *sacredness in the natural, biological order*. . . . He is a person who within the ambience of the flesh claims our care. . . . He is therefore a sacredness in illness and in his dying. . . . The sanctity of human life prevents ultimate trespass upon him even for the sake of treating his bodily life, or for the sake of others who are also only a sacredness in their bodily lives."

18. *Griswold v. Connecticut*, 381 U.S. 479 (1965).

19. *In re Quinlan*, at 665.

20. *In re Quinlan*, at 671.

21. *In re Quinlan*, at 663–64.

22. *In re Quinlan*, at 653.

23. Mrs. Joseph Quinlan, personal communication with Bruce Jennings, April 12, 1996.

24. *In re Quinlan*, at 658–59.

25. *In re Quinlan*, at 664.

26. Michael Oakeshott, "The Voice of Poetry in the Conversation of Mankind," in *Rationalism in Politics and Other Essays* (Indianapolis, Ind.: Liberty Press, 1991).

Chapter 13. Beyond Autonomy

1. Sheldon W. Wolin, *Tocqueville Between Two Worlds: The Making of a Political and Theoretical Life* (Princeton, N.J.: Princeton University Press, 2001).

2. James Madison, *The Federalist*, No. 10, ed. Jacob E. Cooke (Middletown, Conn.: Wesleyan University Press, 1961), 58.

3. John Stuart Mill, *On Liberty* (Indianapolis, Ind.: Bobbs-Merrill, 1956), 13.

4. Reinhold Niebuhr, *The Children of Light and the Children of Darkness* (New York: Charles Scribner's Sons, 1944), 3.

5. Aristotle, *Politics* 1283b–84a, in *The Politics of Aristotle*, ed. and trans. Ernest Barker (NewYork: Oxford University Press, 1971), 134.

6. Daniel Callahan, "Minimalist Ethics" in Arthur Caplan and Daniel Callahan, eds., *Ethics in Hard Times* (New York: Plenum Press, 1981), 261–81.

7. Robert Frost, "Mending Wall," from *North of Boston*, in *Collected Poems, Prose, and Plays*, ed. Richard Poirier and Mark Richardson (New York: Library of America, 1995), 39–40.

8. Gordon S. Wood, *The Radicalism of the American Revolution* (New York: Vintage Books, 1991), 369.

9. Václav Havel, *Open Letters: Selected Writings 1965–1990* (New York: Alfred A. Knopf, 1991), 214.

Index